Traditional Chinese Therapeu

CW00546853

KEEP...
THE CHINESE WAY

Compiled by Hu Bin
Translated by Cai Jingfeng

FOREIGN LANGUAGES PRESS   BEIJING

First Edition 1991
Second Printing 1995

ISBN 7-119-00908-7

© Foreign Languages Press, Beijing, China, 1991

Published by Foreign Languages Press
24 Baiwanzhuang Road, Beijing 100037, China

Distributed by China International Book Trading Corporation
35 Chegongzhuang Xilu, Beijing 100044, China
P.O. Box 399, Beijing, China

Contents

Foreword

Traditional rehabilitation therapy is a time-honoured (going back some two thousand years) system that uses a variety of methods, including breathing exercises, martial arts, massage, acupuncture-moxibustion, chiropractic, slapping, cupping and bloodletting. An important part of China's civilization, it conquers disease and restores health. Its features are:

1. Treatment and prophylaxis of disease, restoration of health and prolongation of life. It is good for the rehabilitation of internal, surgical, gynecological and ophthalmological diseases and is especially useful in conquering diseases most detrimental to human health, such as high blood pressure, arteriosclerotic heart disease, malignancy, pulmonary tuberculosis, liver cirrhosis, chronic nephritis, peptic ulcer and neurosis.

2. This rehabilitation method is also good for curing acute stages of diseases such as acute hepatitis and acute nephritis.

3. It can be used without special medical apparatus or medicament (except necessary adjuvant drugs). The patient feels no uneasiness and experiences no unpleasant reaction; instead, he is relaxed and comfortable during the treatment.

It is therefore a worthwhile therapy for clinical treatment, for maintaining good health and for achieving longevity.

From his own experience, gained through years of practice, and that of others the author hopes to present therapeutic rehabilitation methods to readers in simple, easily understood terms.

Chapter I
Breathing Exercises

Origin and Evolution

Qigong, or breathing exercises, called *daoyin* (directing extremities), *tuna* (exhalation and inhalation) and *lianqi* (training of vital energy) in ancient China, is integral to the search for longevity, a method for keeping fit, strengthening body resistance, and preventing and curing diseases, as well as an important part of rehabilitation medicine. *Qi* (vital energy), refers to the air breathed in and to the "original" *qi** within the body. Practice has shown that strong original *qi* is the vital fundamental factor in conquering diseases and achieving good health, hence traditional Chinese medicine (TCM) stresses training to strengthen original *qi* and its cultivation.

Breathing exercises have a long history of more than twenty-three hundred years. In *The Yellow Emperor's Canon of Internal Medicine,* the earliest extant medical work, written in the Warring States Period in the

---

*Original, genuine, and spiritual *qi* are all special terms in traditional Chinese medicine. Original *qi*, formed in the embryo, is the vital energy responsible for supporting tissues and maintaining physiological functions of the organs. Genuine *qi* is the vital energy located in the kidneys, while spiritual *qi*, also called positive *qi*, is the resistant energy of the body.

fourth century B.C., an entry on breathing exercises reads, "When one is completely at ease, free of desire and ambition, one will get the genuine energy in order and one's mind concentrated, how can diseases invade one's beings? "One must breathe the spiritual energy by concentrating one's mind and relaxing one's muscles." The famous clinician of the Later Han Dynasty Zhang Zhongjing maintained in his *Synopsis of the Golden Cabinet* to treat diseases by *daoyin* and massage. Hua Tuo of the same period (?-298) created the five-animal exercises, the earliest systemic method of *daoyin* training. Cao Yuanfang of the Sui Dynasty recorded in his *Treatise on the Etiology and Symptomatology of Diseases* (published in 610) a great variety of *daoyin* activities. In *Documents of Yimen* Sun Simiao (581-682) of the Tang Dynasty composed a "Song of Hygiene" that reads, "Breathing exercises make the eyesight clear in spring, strengthen the heart in summer, reinforce the lungs in autumn and tone up the kidney in winter. Constant breathing exercises expel evil fever in the *san jiao** and improve digestive functioning." In the Song Dynasty Zhu Xi (1130-1200) directed in his *Maxim for Breathing Exercises*, "Concentrate the mind on the tip of your nose. Relax all parts of your body. Exhale at the end of extreme quietness just like fish swimming in the spring, then inhale like a hibernated worm." This vividly depicts the comfortable sensation after meditation in breathing exercises. The famous doctor of the Jin Dynasty Zhang

---

*San jiao is a general term applied to the organs and tissues located in the thorax, upper abdomen and lower abdomen.

Zihe (c. 1156-1228) also treated diseases through *daoyin* and massage, while Zhu Danxi (1281-1358) of the Yuan Dynasty suggested, "seeking quietness by getting rid of desires," as the theoretical basis for quiet breathing exercises. The distinguished naturalist of the Ming Dynasty Li Shizhen (1518-1593) wrote in his famous work *Encyclopedia of Chinese Materia Medica,* "The channel and collateral system within the body can be perceived only by one who masters the art of breathing." This incisively tells the relationship between the body's channels and breathing exercises. The "theory of quietness" proposed by Wu Shangxian (1806-1886) of the Qing Dynasty could be looked upon as a kind of quiet breathing exercise, while Wang Ren'an (1615-?) of the same dynasty described breathing exercises and methods for seeking longevity from Buddhist and Taoist schools in his *Convalescence Without Medication.* The famous modern physician Zhang Xichun (1860-1933) introduced treatment for seminal emission through breathing exercises in his *Records on Combining Chinese Traditional and Western Medicine.* After the founding of the People's Republic of China breathing exercises were explored thoroughly. Through clinical observation and scientific experiment their effect on high blood pressure, coronary heart disease, peptic ulcers, gastroptosis, neurasthenia and cancer proved satisfactory. Comprehensive breath therapy was applied in many medical institutions nationwide, achieving good results to varying degrees.

Today there is new progress in the study of breathing exercises. For instance, seventeen units, including the Institute of Atomic Energy of the Chinese Academy of

3

Natural Sciences, experimented with the physical and physiological effects of breathing exercises on different individuals some thousand times. They were able to prove that during the course of exercising the individual manifests a series of physical and physiological phenomena different from those of non-exercising individual. Some effects can be detected by modern instruments. This points definitely to the objective presence of *qi* on a substantial basis. Study of the nature of *qi* will ultimately promote research in the life sciences, physics, chemistry and mathematics. Meanwhile it will open a new field in the further development of medical engineering, bionics, the integration of TCM and Western medicine, and the theory of traditional Chinese medicine.

Since the seventies not a few foreign research units have carried out research on breathing exercises, body channels and the nature of *qi* in a multidisciplinary and comprehensive way. International symposia on breathing exercises have been held in Prague, Morocco and Toronto since 1973. In 1975 the Marsh European University in Switzerland made a comprehensive study of breathing exercises from a physiological, biochemical and psychological standpoint. Some three thousand students have graduated from that university, publishing research papers. In 1976 a journal, *Biofeedback,* published in the United States, did a special study on *qigong.* Research societies have been established in Europe, Asia, and North and South America.

Effects

Through his own effort in performing breathing exercises the patient's body functions are regulated achieving muscle relaxation, mental quietude and spiritual stability. On this basis one carries out breathing exercises. It is necessary to control one's mental activities and emotional reactions to arrive at an extremely comfortable and quiet state. This is a kind of therapy for conquering disease and achieving recovery by bringing one's own subjective initiative into full play and strengthening body resistance.

The three integral parts of breathing exercises are adjusting the body (posture), adjusting the mind (meditation) and adjusting the respiration (breathing). All these parts act on the body as a whole. All research on breathing exercises has proved their definite and positive effect on each organ and system of the body.

(1) Effect on the Nervous System

During the exercise the nervous system is in a state of internal inhibition due to mental quietness. Experience and study have proved that quietness eliminates tension in the cerebral cortex, reinforces its adjusting capacity and improves the functions of all body organs.

Comprehensive study by scientists found that the electroencephalographic waves from various parts of the cortex were different in their voltage, but their amplitude didn't exceed 50 microvolts. After breathing exercises the voltage increased to as much as 150 to 180 microvolts, with synchronous increase in electroencephalogram voltage in all areas of the cortex. The better the mastery of the exercise, the higher the synchronism. This shows that breathing exercises will bring the electric activity of the nerve cells to a high degree of orderliness, resulting in low consumption and high efficacy of the brain.

Experiments also revealed that after exercising, patients with high blood pressure showed a relative weakening of reaction in the sympathetic nerve, while that of the parasympathetic nerve was strengthened. Also, the activity of dopa-B-hydroxylase was lowered— another sign of the weakening excitation in the sympathetic nerve.

Breath therapy is different from sleep therapy in that it arouses the patient's own subjective initiative, controlling nervous activity. It is not a dormant state but a state "completely free of desire and ambition" and a "concentration of the mind." Such a condition exerts obvious protective actions and is beneficial to the active rest of the cortex.

(2) Effect on the Cardiovascular System

Breathing exercises promote blood circulation by dilating the capillaries and strengthening the pulse. The patient's heartbeat slows down after exercise, with an increase in cardiac output when inhaling deeply and an increase in returning blood volume during deep exhaling. The burden of the heart can be lightened through breathing exercises so sufferers of hypertension and arteriosclerosis will suffer no further hypertrophy or enlargement of their hearts. During exercise the patient experiences meditation by focusing his consciousness on a certain site, for instance the lower *dan tian** (the umbilicus or *qihai* point) or upper *dan tian* (*yintang* or *baihui* point). His blood pressure decreases or increases respectively. From an electrocardiogram it can be seen that the exerciser's heartbeat slows down markedly, with recovery from arrhythmia after exercise. His heart burden is thus lessened resulting in decreased oxygen consumption and strengthened cardiac functions.

(3) Effect on the Digestive System

During abdominal breathing in *qigong*, when using the counterbreath method or the breath-holding method organs in the abdominal cavity seem to be massaged rhythmically. The diaphragm's range of movement is three or four times that during regular breathing. The rhythmic change of intra-abdominal pressure "massages" the stomach, intestines, liver, gallbladder and pancreas, causing an increase of gastrointestinal peristalsis and thus of juice secretion and a decrease of abdominal blood stagnation, improving digestion and absorption functions. Exercising promotes good appetite, complete assimilation and gain in body weight. Under X-ray examination the tension of the gastrointestinal tract is seen to increase with active and rhythmic peristalsis. As soon as the exercising begins, the breath frequency starts to lower down gradually,

---

Dan tian: site in the human body as denoted in TCM. The midpoint between the umbilicus and the *qihai* point is called lower *dan tian*, the point at the centre of the epigastrium is called intermediate *dan tian*. The midpoint between *yintang* (the midpoint between the two eyebrows) and *baihui* is called upper *dan tian*. *Qihai*, *yintang* and *baihui* are all acupoints. Generally the term *dan tian* refers to lower *dan tian* unless there is a clear indication that upper or intermediate *dan tian* is meant.

with an ever louder, ever more frequent gurgling sound in the intestines. After exercising, these changes revert to normal. Since movements of the gastrointestinal tract are controlled by the sympathetic nervous system, the excitation of the nervus vagus is also strengthened. This markedly improves the function of the digestive system.

(4) Effect on the Respiratory System

After long observation it can be seen that the physical effect during exercising is rather remarkable. When an expert in breathing exercises is functioning, a periodically induced signal of 30 mv can be detected even when his fingers are 30 cm away from the voltage meter, whereas a layman or an exerciser not yet fully functioning shows no electric change. This demonstrates that the electromagnetic field around a functioning expert is quite different from that of a nonexerciser or an exerciser not yet functioning. This phenomenon is called emission of internal energy. In abdominal breathing the amplitude of the diaphragm's movement is three to four times that in regular breathing, and breath frequency and ventilation volume per minute decrease. Meanwhile, oxygen consumption decreases 30 percent compared with that prior to exercising. Metabolic rate decreases 20 percent. These changes are termed a low metabolic, physiological state, which is helpful to decrease body expenditure so as to build up body resistance for conquering disease and to regain health.

(5) Effect on the Endocrine System

The cerebral cortex is in a state of inhibition when

the exerciser achieves meditation or quietness. The endocrine glands, being closely linked with one another, are under the control of the nervous system and function as one system, hence their secretions (hormones) can be kept in either synergistic or antagonistic condition in line with the demand of the organism. Hyperfunction will result from the case of excessive secretion and vice versa— both abnormal. With apparent lower metabolic rate the oxygen consumption of an expert exerciser is 16 percent lower than that of a normal individual when awake, who, asleep, consumes only 10 percent less oxygen than when awake. It has been demonstrated by measuring the biochemical change of central nerve mediator that the metabolism of 5-hydroxy tryptamine in an exerciser has a level one to two times higher than that in a normal individual, while that of adrenaline and noradrenaline are much lower, only 60 percent of the normal rate. That is one reason an exerciser enjoys comfort and relaxation. Breathing exercises also lessen the secretions of corticohormones and growth hormones, causing a slow turnover rate of protein, changes in enzymatic activity and strengthening of the body's immunity.

(6) Summary

From the above descriptions it is clear that breathing exercises can prevent and treat disease, prolong life and reinforce body resistance. Though the nature of these exercises is still far from thoroughly understood, they are based on firm scientific ground. Practice has proved that breathing exercises induce a metabolic balance more appropriate to living. This may be the basis for rehabilitation and strengthening of body resistance.

In TCM *qi* (vital energy) does possess a substantial basis. By imitating the physical effects induced by breathing exercises, man has begun to make medical instruments that will enable this time-honoured art to make new contributions to the health of mankind.

Methods

(1) Adjusting the Body (Posture)

Correct posture is the first step in breathing exercises. Natural relaxation of all your muscles is a prerequisite for successful execution of breathing exercises and the inducement of mental relaxation and quietness. Various postures possess different physiological features, and posture itself plays an indisputable role in the elimination of disease. The postures commonly adopted are normal sitting, natural cross-legged, single cross-legged, supine, lying on side, standing and walking postures.

1. Normal sitting posture (Fig. 1): Sit upright on a square stool with the feet touching the ground, the legs apart, and the knees bent at right angles. Put hands naturally on knees or make fists in front of lower abdomen. Retract chin naturally, drop shoulders and relax chest. Close the eyes and mouth, letting the tip of the tongue touch the hard palate. Smile.

2. Natural cross-legged posture (Fig. 2): Sit upright on a "8" plank bed or bench with the legs crossed to form the letter. Rest hands in front of lower abdomen or on knees.

3. Single cross-legged posture (Fig. 3): Sit upright on

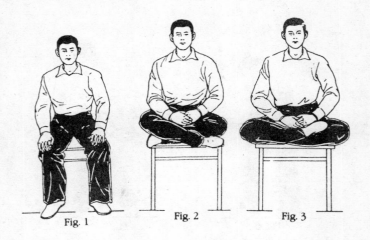

Fig. 1   Fig. 2   Fig. 3

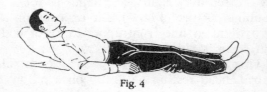

Fig. 4

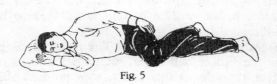

Fig. 5

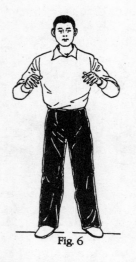

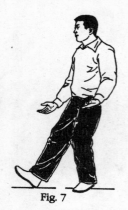

Fig. 6   Fig. 7

a plank bed or bench with right leg crossed over left or left leg crossed over right. Rest hands as for 2.

4. Supine posture (Fig. 4): Lie on back on a plank bed at a slight incline from upper to lower body, legs straight, arms at sides.

5. Lying on side posture (Fig. 5): Lie on side on a plank bed, head resting naturally on a pillow. Upper half of body is straight, with upper leg bent over lower and upper hand on buttock. Put lower hand on pillow in front with palm upward. Patient may lie on left or right side, but a cardiac patient is advised to lie on right side.

6. Standing posture (Fig. 6): The most popular posture is the "three-ball style." Patient stands straight with feet shoulder width apart, toes pointed slightly inward and knees slightly bent. Relax chest and raise

arms until elbows are slightly lower than shoulders, the hands being 33 cm apart and as if holding a big ball; each hand is curved as if holding a small ball. Eyes and mouth are shut gently and exerciser smiles slightly.

7. Walking posture (Fig. 7): After standing quietly two to three minutes, the exerciser steps forward, the left heel touching the ground first and trunk and hands swinging towards the right. Exhale through the mouth, inhale through the nose. As soon as the left sole touches the ground completely, the right foot steps forward in like manner and trunk and hands swing to the opposite side. The exerciser thus walks forward step by step. The duration of each practice session depends on one's condition and capacity. Generally it lasts half an hour.

(2) Adjusting the Mind (Meditation)

Adjusting the mind to get into a state of quietness is fundamental to breathing exercises. The effect of the exercise is determined primarily by the degree of meditation. The deeper one gets into it, the greater the therapeutic effect (the exerciser must maintain stable quietness without any distracting thought). Meditation refers to concentration of the mind on a certain point, such as *dan tian*, or on one's respiration. Perception of external stimuli is greatly attenuated, even to loss of orientation or sensation of body weight—a protective inhibition of the cerebral cortex. There are five ways to get into such a state:

1. Point concentration: The mind is strongly concentrated on a certain point in the body, usually the *dan tian* point (just below the umbilicus). The exerciser should be free of all distracting thoughts. However, this need not be taken too seriously, so long as one is in a

state of natural quietness and concentrate oneself to an appropriate degree.

2. Free breathing: Concentrate on the in and out movements of the abdomen as you breathe. However, do not direct the movements consciously, so that you can reach a state of quietness and natural unity of breath and mind.

3. Counting while breathing: In Chinese one round of respiration, i.e. exhalation and inhalation, is called *xi*. During exercise, count your *xi* silently from one to ten, to one hundred, until you reach a state of seeing nothing, hearing nothing, thinking nothing, thus quite naturally arriving at meditation.

4. Reading silently: The reading matter should be as simple as possible, so that all distracting thoughts are replaced by a single thought to achieve meditation. For instance, just read silently the two words *silence* and *relaxation*. Quite a few people are able to get into a state free of distracting thoughts—carefree, joyous, comfortable and sedate.

5. Listening to the breaths: Concentrate on the sound of your own breath. However, it is better to hear nothing, in order to get into meditation.

A beginner should choose the first method, then proceed gradually to the second or fifth method. Or choose any one of the five methods and stick to it.

(3) Adjusting the Respiration (Breathing)

Breathing is a key link in *qigong* therapy. Through conscious exercise it can be changed from the usual thoracic type to an abdominal type, from shallow to deep breathing, and eventually to a *dan tian* type (lower abdominal type).* As a result, the vital capacity is increased; the gas metabolism and blood circulation are improved, and the "massage" of the internal viscerae promotes food digestion and absorption. All these changes strengthen the body, preventing and curing diseases.

The eight common types of breathing are:

1. Natural breathing: This is an instinct that needs no conscious control. The movements are gentle, smooth, even and natural. However, it has the drawback of shallowness and short duration.

2. Harmonious breathing: The diaphragm descends and the abdominal wall protrudes during inhalation; the reverse occurs during exhalation. It should be exercised to achieve great amplitude of diaphragmatic movements and the abdominal wall, leading to the abdominal type of breathing.

3. Reverse breathing: The movements of the diaphragm and abdominal wall are just the reverse of those for harmonious breathing. The amplitude and force of the movements are also greater.

4. Hold breath: There are two types; one prolongs the period between the inhalation and exhalation (inhalation-hold breath-exhalation), while the other

---

*Ancient medical literature describes the sensation experienced by *qigong* experts as that the vital energy sinking into the *dan tian* during deep breathing. This is, of course, an archaic hypothesis. In fact, the sensation comes from a natural protrusion of the abdominal wall as a result of increased pressure caused by the movement of the diaphragm during respiration. Air can enter only the lungs through the nostrils or mouth; outside air cannot enter the abdomen. From a scientific viewpoint *dan tian* breathing refers to the subjective sensation during deep breathing when the diaphragm descends and the lower abdomen protrudes as if air were entering the abdomen.

prolongs the period between the exhalation and inhalation (inhalation-exhalation-hold breath).

5. Nasal inhalation, oral exhalation: This type of breathing is used when the nasal, or upper respiratory, passages are obstructed.

6. Ventilation through the *du* and *ren* channels: The exerciser inhales through the nose, then imagines that the air (*qi*, or vital energy) is being directed to his umbilicus and on to his perineum. After that, he imagines that the air passes from the perineum through the spinal column to the *baihui* point at the top of the head (the apex), to be exhaled through the nose. This is termed the "lesser respiratory cycle" of breathing.

7. Latent breathing: This kind of breathing occurs naturally after practising harmonious or reverse breathing. It consists of soft inhalation and exhalation in a smooth cycle. A finger under the exerciser's nostrils will detect no obvious air.

8. True breath: There is an old Chinese saying: "Ordinary breathing eventually comes to an end, but true breathing doesn't." The stopping of the breath doesn't mean a forced stopping, but the spontaneous result of an extreme quietness of the mind. The quieter the mind, the softer the breath. The vital energy seems to cease and the mind seems "frozen"; only a very slight breath signifies the presence of life. Superficially, the exerciser seems to stop breathing, but actually he is still breathing through his umbilicus. That is called "foetal breathing," an advanced stage in breathing exercises.

Of the above methods, the harmonious and reverse breathing methods are good for preventing and curing cardiovascular and cerebralvascular diseases; held breath is good for preventing and curing digestive diseases; nasal inhalation, oral exhalation for respiratory diseases; ventilation through the *du* and *ren* channels for the nervous system. It is advisable for patients to choose the method best suited to their condition and disease, in order to avoid error. However, whatever method you choose, you should revert to normal breathing after ten to twenty minutes' exercise; otherwise the respiratory muscles will be strained, resulting in dyspnea and paralysis. To avoid such a turn, a combination of breathing exercise and rest is necessary. The exerciser shouldn't be overanxious for quick results; instead he should proceed step by step, following the basic rules to achieve smooth, deep, even and gentle breathing.

Types of Breathing Exercises

The methods for practice have just been introduced. However, there are different types of breathing exercises. Here the commonly most effective ones are introduced for selection.

(1) Quiet, Relaxed Exercise
The sequence of quiet, relaxed breathing exercise is preparation, posture, relaxation, breathing, sitting quietly, ending.

1. Preparation
In breathing exercises the main object is to achieve deep quietude of the cerebral cortex through adjusting the mind and vital energy. As a rule, the exerciser is full of distracting thoughts and finds it hard to concen-

trate in order to reach a state of quietude. A preparatory period is necessary to eliminate all disturbances and ensure the success of the breathing exercise.

(a) Choose a quiet, clean environment, indoors or outdoors, with fresh air and good ventilation, but do not exercise in a direct draught, to avoid catching cold.

(b) Whatever position you adopt —lying, standing, sitting or walking— buttons, belt, shoelaces and tight clothing should be all loosened to facilitate blood circulation and ease the body.

(c) Rest twenty minutes to stabilize your mood before exercising. Thus, your mind can easily concentrate with happy feelings. If you are in an unstable, rash mood with distracting thoughts and your respiration is not smooth, it is difficult to achieve quietude. If you are dispirited you will soon fall asleep and the effect will be unsatisfactory.

2. Assuming your posture

Whatever posture you select, a right, natural posture is essential to get into quietude. A wide stool or chair should be equal in height to the length of your legs from the knees down. The head, neck and trunk should be erect, the head inclined forward slightly, the buttocks protruding backward a little. Don't expand the chest or bend the back. In cross-legged posture put one hand over the other with the palms facing upward or clasp the fingers of one hand with the other; put hands on legs or just in front of the lower abdomen. Gently close your eyes by gazing at your own nose; the tip of the tongue should lightly touch the hard palate.

3. Relaxation

Relaxation, essential for all breathing exercises, aims at the elimination of all mental tension and complete relaxation of all the muscles, viscera, vessels and nerves so as to achieve a state of natural comfort with the vital energy sinking into *dan tian.*

Whatever the posture, relaxation should begin at the head and work towards the feet. The head is "pushed" upward very gently, the shoulders are relaxed and dropped naturally. The chest and abdomen are both relaxed without protrusion. The mind is completely without tension, and the face is smiling.

4. Breathing

We have just explained that the different types of breathing meet the needs of various diseases and physiques. Therefore, selecting the correct breathing method, according to the individual, disease and condition, is essential for the active therapeutic effect of breathing exercises.

For the quiet, relaxed breathing exercise harmonious breathing is used; silently say the word *quietness* during inhalation and the word *relaxation* during exhalation. The better you relax, the sooner you can get into quietness. Respiration should be natural, gentle and comfortable, with the vital energy sunk into the *dan tian*, reaching the state of "returning every breath to its root source." Since breathing practice is the key link in breathing exercises, it is necessary to practise conscientiously. Without proper breathing there will be no therapeutic effect. Nevertheless, you must not get overanxious about success. Instead, you should approach the goal step by step. Twenty to thirty minutes for each practice session is sufficient. Practice should be combined with rest so as to avoid any ill effects from excessive practice.

5. Sitting quietly

Learning to sit quietly should follow breath training. In the beginning distracting thoughts are apt to disturb your concentration. By concentrating on *dan tian*, you will ultimately eliminate such thoughts. If distracting thoughts cannot be eliminated, you might try the method of listening to your breath. "Listening" doesn't mean to listen to the sound of your breath, but to pay attention to the whereabouts of each inhalation and exhalation. It is not necessary to pay attention to the frequency, quality and depth of the breathing. Distracting thoughts will disappear completely, and you will be in meditation. The degree of meditation varies with different individuals and different diseases and can't be sought reluctantly or forced. The more anxious you are, the more difficult it will be for you to reach such a state, for impatience itself is the result of distracting thoughts that prevent the attainment of quietude, a state that can be entered only through patient and gradual practice. However, since quietude is a relative state, it is unreasonable for the beginner to seek deep quietude. Even though you are not reaching a satisfactory state of quietude, substituting concentration on a single thought for distracting thoughts, you can still experience the therapeutic effect to some degree.

6. Ending

At the end of the exercise don't get up hurriedly. Press your umbilicus with one palm over the back of the other palm, then massage gently, the umbilicus moving around in a circle from small to large clockwise for about thirty cycles, followed by a reverse movement—from large circle to small anticlockwise for another thirty cycles.

7. Effective for: hypertension, hypertensive heart disease, arteriosclerotic coronary disease, rheumatic heart disease, cor pulmonale, rheumatic arthritis, chronic bronchitis, emphysema, pulmonary cancer, bronchiectasis, bronchia asthma, peptic ulcer, chronic gastritis, chronic enteritis, chronic pancreatitis, stomach cancer, esophageal cancer, chronic nephritis, chronic pyelonephritis, neurasthenia, neurosis, chronic hepatitis, adipose liver, cerebral arteriosclerosis, rheumatoid arthritis, etc.

8. Contraindications: schizophrenia, melancholia, hysteria, hyperpyrexia, massive hemorrhage, etc.

(2) Internal Healing Exercise

1. Preparatory work same as above.

2. Posture same as above.

3. Physical and mental conditions should be relaxed, without any tension and natural.

4. Held breath is adopted for this exercise. There are two types: inhale, hold breath, exhale, inhale; inhale, exhale, hold breath, inhale. These movements are repeated over and over again. In each session the breathing should be smooth and gentle and attention should be paid to the following:

(a) Respiration should be deep, long, gentle, smooth and even. During the whole process inhalation should be gentle and slight so as to produce a deep, long, noiseless breath. Unless the breathing is gentle and smooth, the exercise can't last long. Inhalation, hold, exhalation should be even and should not be pushed to their limits. Only in this way can the respiration be kept stable. To test whether the breathing accords with demand, one simply listens. A noiseless breath is satisfactory.

(b) Establish a conditioned reflex of inhalation and exhalation through the nostrils and direct the vital energy to sink to the *dan tian*. This can be accomplished by consciously inducing the sensation of air descending towards the lower abdomen (just below the navel) during breathing, and it can be established within a fairly short period. Some exercisers might be overanxious to achieve such a conditioned reflex and force the abdominal wall out (by simply moving abdominal muscles), hold the breath, etc. This would result in thoracic respiration, in which the diaphragm descends only a short distance or even not at all and the vital energy can't reach as far down as the *dan tian* level. Moreover, the exerciser's upper body moves up and down with the respiratory movements, so it is easy to get exhausted and not be able to continue. Hence, the exerciser must have patience in cultivating such a conditioned reflex.

(c) Hold breath. The passage of vital energy and expansion of the abdomen are gradually and naturally achieved through practice. The extent of expansion and retraction of the abdominal wall varies with different individuals and different stages of practice. It is a misunderstanding that the lower abdomen should be made to protrude as far as possible. The exerciser is apt to become exhausted and certain complaints are likely to occur. Therefore, forced tension should be avoided.

5. Concentration on the *dan tian* is one of the key links in breathing exercises. The aim is to focus the mind, get rid of all distractions and hold to a single thought so as to achieve complete tranquillity of the brain. The calmer the brain, the greater the therapeutic

effect. A satisfactory condition for the brain is a stable, quiet, semisleeping state in which the highest nerve centre reaches a protective inhibitory effect, which, together with the advantageous activity of the internal organs, eventually results in normal physiological functions of the body. During breathing practice, one should carefully experience one's own natural, gentle, stable and comfortable respiration and concentrate one's mind. This facilitates gaining tranquillity.

It is not easy immediately to get rid of distractions, for in the beginning the cerebral cortex has not yet entered a quiet state. A conditioned reflex for getting rid of distracting thoughts can be established only through persistent practice.

Pure thought without distraction is prerequisite for tranquillity, which in ancient times was called "adjusting the mind," meaning to transform distracting thoughts into the single thought of quietude. Generally, this goes along with adjusting the breathing. Counting the breath, tracking the breath, holding the breath, observing the breath, returning the breath and quiet breathing are all beneficial to combining vital energy and consciousness. Counting means to count silently the frequency of the breath; tracking means to follow the breath consciously; holding means that the breath seems to be stopping at the *dan tian*; observing means "viewing" from the inside as the breath moves gently through the nostrils; returning means breathing completely unconsciously; quiet breathing means the exerciser is totally free of distraction, clear and silent, with the mind as quiet as a pool of still water. All these methods facilitate reaching tranquillity. Any one or two, such as tracking or holding the breath or quiet breathing, will prove excellent. Only through conscientious practice can the body probe the depths.

6. Ending same as previous description.

7. Effective for: Chronic gastritis, peptic ulcer of stomach and duodenum, gastroptosis, dyspepsia, chronic hepatitis, chronic cholecystitis, allergic colitis, chronic pancreatitis, chronic enteritis, chronic appendicitis, chronic colitis, adipose liver, habitual constipation, etc. In carcinoma of stomach, intestine and mammary glands it might serve as a subsidiary treatment.

8.Contraindications: pulmonary tuberculosis (cavity type), bronchiectasis, pulmonary emphysema (incorrect use of held breath might lead to massive hemoptysis caused by rupture of vessels in the cavities and bronchioles), peptic ulcer with strong pisitive test for occult blood, massive hemorrhage in peptic ulcer, hypertension, hypertensive heart disease, cor pulmonale, coronary sclerotic heart disease, rheumatic heart disease, arrhythmia, auricular fibrillation, extrasystole, obstruction of the cardiac conduction system. This exercise would have a harmful effect on these ailments.

(3) Robust Exercise

First of all, the essentials of the exercise should be handled carefully, i.e., correct posture, adjustment of breathing and concentration of the mind on tranquillity.

1. Preparatory procedures same as for quiet, relaxed exercise.

2. Correct posture results in easy quietude. No matter which posture you assume, it must be regular and natural. In sitting posture sit up straight or cross-legged with one leg on the other. If you feel pain or numbness,

just move the lower leg above, or straighten your legs. Resume a cross-legged posture until no numbness is felt.

(a) The head should be upright, the chin retracted, the eyes and mouth closed gently. The tip of the tongue touches the hard palate. The mouth smiles.

(b) The vertebral column should be erect, with the caudal part protruding back slightly and the lumbar vertebra protruding slightly forward. The buttocks rest on a cushion. Don't throw the chest forward. Arms and shoulders drop naturally with the abdomen relaxed. The muscles of the whole body are relaxed without any feeling of binding.

(c) The hands, in a loose fist, are placed in front of the lower abdomen with the four fingers and thumb of one hand grasping those of the other hand. The hands may also rest on the knees.

3. Breathing

At the beginning respiration should conform to individual habit. As a rule, men usually breathe in the "harmonious" way, while women usually breathe in the "reverse" way. For this exercise exercisers should practise the reverse of their habitual pattern. In practising one should rest by adopting natural and habitual respiration after ten to twenty minutes of breathing exercise to avoid side effects due to overfatigue of the respiratory muscles. While exercising, make sure the exhalation is natural and gentle, pay no attention to the inhalation and keep the breathing smooth without any deviation.

4. Sitting quietly

After the breathing exercise you should practise sitting quietly. During respiration concentrating the mind on the respiration will result in a "unity of mind and vital energy," thus making it easy to enter meditation. If you don't do the breathing exercise and simply practise sitting quietly, use the following method to replace distracting thoughts by a single thought, and enter meditation, concentrating on the *dan tian*, listening to the breath, counting the breath and reading silently, then one enters a state of semiconsciousness and self-forgetfulness—just right. Sit quietly for thirty to forty minutes, then move on to the next step.

5. Ending

At the end of sitting quietly one should direct one's vital energy to circle the umbilicus from left to right twenty-four times. Then reverse direction and circle thirty-six times. After that one may leave his seat.

6. Action exercise

In breathing exercises action is less than quietness. Action is mainly practised by the abdominal type of deep breathing in which the movements of the diaphragm and abdominal muscles massage the viscera. This is called internal action. After the breathing exercise traditional Chinese shadow boxing (*taijiquan*), setting-up exercises to music, traditional Chinese eight-part gymnastics, slow running, etc., may be performed. Any one or two activities may be chosen and if performed over a long period will have a satisfactory effect.

7. Effective for: Besides the ailments listed under quiet, relaxed exercise, the following are worth mentioning: neurosis, neurasthenia, functional disorders of the sympathetic nervous system. Robust exercise is particularly good for strengthening somatic power, protecting health and treating and preventing disease.

8. Contraindications same as for previous exercises.

(4) Transmission and Strength-Directing Exercises
Normally seminal emission occurs once every seven to fifteen days in youths. Repeated and uncontrolled emissions within a week denote a pathological condition and should be treated in time, otherwise the condition will eventually lead to exhaustion, dizziness, tinnitus, memory failure, lack of concentration, weakness, palpitations, shortness of breath, backache, pain in the waist or legs, etc., affecting not only one's work but also one's study and health. Emission usually results from overfatigue, extreme mental tension, neurasthenia, too much sleep, unduly soft mattress, prone sleeping posture or the reading of pornographic books and materials. These exercises are designed especially for treating emission.

1. Transmission exercise
(a) Preparation: Loosen the belt and clothing buttons. Evacuate the rectum and bladder. The surroundings should be calm and the air fresh.
(b) Points to remember: The exercise is performed on a bed inclined so that one end is about ten centimetres higher than the other, or the exerciser may sit on his pillow. A wooden plank bed is good. A bed with steel springs or coir ropes is too soft for such an exercise.

The exercise is performed twice daily, before going to bed and just after getting up. Facing the foot of the bed, the exerciser sits with legs extended straight ahead and toes pointed upward. The trunk is upright and the palms cover the kneecaps (Fig. 8). Then the exerciser clenches his fists and draws the elbows back as far as

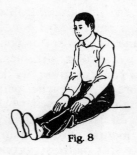

Fig. 8

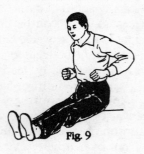

Fig. 9

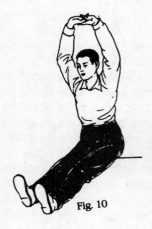

Fig. 10

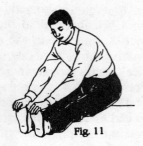

Fig. 11

possible with each fist close to either side (Fig. 9). Loosen the fists with the palms facing upward. The exerciser begins to inhale with the abdominal wall retracted. At the same time he extends his arms upward close to the ears and eventually straightens them just like a weightlifter until he can't extend them any farther. Meanwhile he should elevate and constrict his sphincter muscles, just as if he were blocking an urgent defecation. In that position he interlaces his fingers with palms upward and his eyes gazing at the backs of his hands and begins to exhale (Fig. 10). Then he leans forward to touch his toes (Fig. 11), returning finally to the original position. This completes the exercise. Begin by doing it ten times in succession, then day by day add two rounds, until by the end of the first month you will have added sixty rounds. With the original ten, that makes seventy altogether. Continue without adding any more. After the exercise sit quietly for twenty to thirty minutes.

(c) Some requirements for the transmission exercise

When you are touching the toes with the fingers, the legs should be straight. No bending is permitted. It may be difficult in the beginning, but after persistent effort you will succeed. In extending the arms and facing the palms upward, one must inhale gently and smoothly. Be sure to elevate and constrict the anal muscles when extending the interlaced fingers. When lowering the head and bending the back, one should exhale gently. Finally, sitting quietly to ease the mind is also necessary.

2. Strength-directing exercise

(a) Preparation same as above.

(b) Sit upright on a stool or bed with the chin

slightly retracted, the neck slightly relaxed and bent. The legs may be either extended or crossed. Clench the fists. The mind should be quiet and comfortable and the face smiling. All muscles should be relaxed and the eyes closed gently. The mind is concentrated on the umbilicus. Sit silently for ten to twenty minutes, then start abdominal breathing. During inhalation the shoulders are raised and the neck retracted just as if you were carrying a heavy object on your head. Then elevate and constrict the sphincter muscle as if blocking an urgent defecation, with the abdominal wall retracted inward. During exhalation the movements are reversed. Lower the shoulders slowly. The abdominal wall protrudes gently and naturally. Do these movements twenty times. After that the respiration should be restored to normal. Sit silently for another twenty minutes before standing up. The exercise should be performed twice daily, in the morning after getting up and in the evening before going to bed. Increase the movement cycle by one each day until you reach a total of fifty cycles. Directing one's vital energy, or strength, requires gentle, natural unforced movement. Persevere and the ailment will be cured within two months.

(c) Effective for emission when awake or asleep, and sexual neurasthenia.

(5) *Daoyin* (Ancient Breathing and Physical Exercise)
Daoyin combines breathing exercises with physical exercises. Recently *daoyin* charts were among cultural relics unearthed in the Han tomb of Mawangdui in the suburbs of Changsha, Hunan Province. The charts date back to 186 B.C. and illustrate some forty *daoyin*

postures. Apparently *daoyin* has been a method for keeping fit for two thousand years. One type of *daoyin* is described below.

This *daoyin* exercise is a standing type of breathing exercise in which the vital energy is consciously directed up or down, left or right, to flow freely within the body. The thought directs the *qi*, or vital energy; the *qi* directs the blood circulation. When the exercise is successful, the exerciser feels his vital energy flowing with the rhythm of his respiration. This "inner vital energy" flows along courses corresponding to the diseased viscera or channels. For instance, inner vital energy can be directed to the diseased stomach and concentrated there at the same time, so can it be done to a diseased liver or other viscera. For hypertension an exerciser may direct his inner energy from the upper *dan tian* (located between the eyebrows) to the *yongquan* point (the acupoint at the depression of the anterior sole when retracting the toes) along the *ren* channel at the midline of the chest and abdomen, whereas for hypotension the inner energy may be directed voluntarily in the opposite direction. Constant practice will result in the improvement of blood and lymphatic circulation, adjustment of nerve function, increase in metabolism, increase in tissue and functions of the diseased viscera and enhancement of resilience. Thus the disease will ameliorate and eventually be cured.

1. Preparatory procedures: Loosen clothing. Evacuate the bladder and bowels. Drink a cup of warm water.

2. Relaxation of the muscles: the head is held straight; chest and arms are relaxed. All the body parts, including the waist, shoulders and hips, are

relaxed naturally. One's appearance should be peaceful, happy and smiling.

(a) Stomach exercise 1 (Fig. 12): After the muscles are relaxed, step to the left so feet are shoulder width apart. Raise both hands slowly to shoulder height, then lower slowly. Bend the knees slightly so they are in line with the toes; the hands should be in line with the nipples and as if holding a ball. The mind is concentrated on the *dan tian* and the energy initiates from the Vital Gate (an acupoint between the second and third lumbar vertebrae). During inhalation the abdominal wall protrudes as the waist moves forward, while during exhalation the movements are reversed. In other words, the waist moves forward and backward naturally like a pendulum. After thirty to sixty rounds stand quietly for three to five minutes.

Helpful to digestion, capable of strengthening body resistance.

(b) Kidney exercise (Fig. 13)

Posture: Starting with the above position, put the hands in front of the knees about one Chinese foot (33 cm) apart. Concentrate on the Vital Gate point, then rotate the trunk at the waist from left to right thirty-six times and from right to left twenty-four times. Stand quietly three to five minutes. The circular movement should be small, round, gentle, natural and smooth.

For curing waist pain, increasing physical strength.

(c) Depressor exercise (Fig. 14)

Posture: Starting with the same posture, put hands about five Chinese inches (16 cm) beside hips naturally. The body is thus in a bell-shaped position. Then the lower extremities tremble slightly, moving upward until the whole body is trembling and relaxed. The exer-

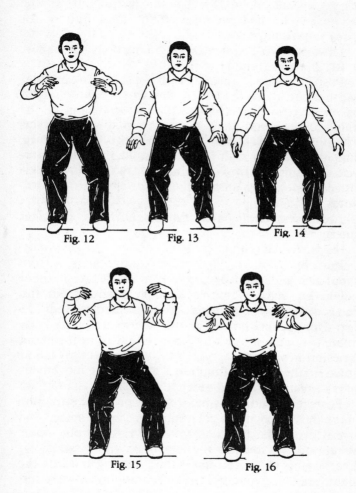

Fig. 12　　　　Fig. 13　　　　Fig. 14

Fig. 15　　　　Fig. 16

33

ciser feels his blood flowing downward. Sustain the movement for two minutes, then stand quietly for three to five minutes.

Lowers blood pressure, strengthens body resistance.

(d) Lung exercise (Fig. 15)

Posture: Stand upright with legs about shoulder width apart. Raise the hands slowly to shoulder height, then each forms a circle. Use reverse breathing, i.e. the diaphragm ascends and the abdominal wall retracts when inhaling, descends and protrudes when exhaling. The air flows through the nostrils. The mind concentrates on the *dan tian* (umbilicus). Do the movements fifteen times, then stand quietly for three to five minutes.

Increases vital capacity, strengthens physical strength.

(e) Heart exercise (Fig. 16)

Posture: Standing as before, move hands from shoulders and each arm makes a circle at shoulder height. Use natural respiration. The mind concentrates on the *tanzhong* point (an acupoint located between the two nipples, on the midline of the chest). The body doesn't move but stays in a relaxed position for about five minutes.

Strengthens heart function.

(f) Liver and spleen exercise (Fig. 17)

Posture: Standing as before, move the arms akimbo and hands to positions corresponding to the spleen and liver. Swing the trunk to left and right at the waist. When moving towards the left, press and massage the liver region with the right palm; moving towards the right, press and massage the spleen region with the left palm. Do the movement fifteen times each. Movements should be gentle, even, comfortable and smooth, with the mind concentrated on the *dan tian*.

Improves blood circulation, increases physical strength.

(g) Opening the *du* and *ren* channels (Fig. 18)

Posture: Stand upright with feet shoulder width apart. Eyes gaze forward with the mind concentrated. Raise arms gradually to shoulder height and chest width. Flex knees slightly and crouch down with the mind concentrating on the *dan tian*. The vital energy is directed by the mind; air is inhaled through the nose to the umbilicus, to the *qihai* (five centimetres below the umbilicus), to the perineum(between the anus and scrotum or vulva); pause a moment, then exhale the air from the perineum to the coccyx and along the spine to the *yuzhen* point (a little above the external occipital protuberance of the occipital bone), to the upper *dan tian* and out the nostrils. Do the cycle three times, then stand quietly for three to five minutes.

Harmonizes the *yin-yang* principles of the body and strengthens the body.

(h) Closing the *dai* channel (Fig. 19)

Posture: Standing as before, extend the arms sideways at shoulder height, palms upward. The mind concentrates on the *dan tian*. The air inhaled, directed by the mind, starts from the *dan tian* and circles the waist to the left once, then exhales the air circling once to the right. Do ten times.

Cures abdominal distention and strengthens the body.

(i) Pressing the *weizhong* point (Fig. 20)

Posture: Standing as before, extend the arms sideways to form a 45-degree angle with the trunk. Move

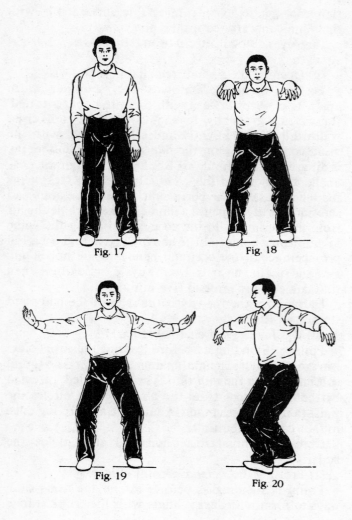

Fig. 17

Fig. 18

Fig. 19

Fig. 20

right foot and trunk obliquely to the right. Flex the right knee, then turn the left toe in and bring the left leg behind so that the left knee presses against the *weizhong* point at the back of the right knee. Then press the *weizhong* point at the back of the left knee. Do ten times on each side.

Effective for waist pain and backache.

(j) *Yin-yang* toe-tip tap (Fig. 21)

Posture: Stand upright. Turn the body obliquely to the left. Flex the left knee slightly and shift body weight to the left leg. Tap the ground with the right toe tip. Separate the hands and put them beside the hips. Press hands downward. Concentrate on the *dan tian*. During inhalation the air is directed down the outside of the thigh to the *yongquan* point on the sole of the foot; during exhalation returns to the *dan tian* along the inside of the thigh. Do the movements five times for each foot.

Makes the legs nimble.

(k) The *yin-yang* heel tap (Fig. 22)

Posture: Standing, turn to the right obliquely. Flex the left leg to support the body weight. Extend the right foot forward with the heel touching the ground, the toes pointing upward. Put the hands on each side of the abdomen with palms upward. Concentrate on the central part of the chest, between the nipples. During inhalation direct the air from this point along the outside of the arms to the palms; during exhalation direct the air back along the inside of the arms. Do the exercise five times on each side.

Cures stomachache and heart pain.

(l) Balancing exercise (Fig. 23)

Posture: Standing as before, turn the body obliquely

37

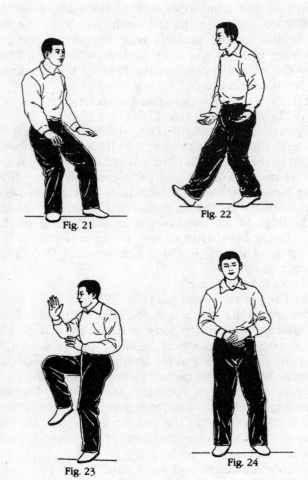

Fig. 21

Fig. 22

Fig. 23

Fig. 24

to the left. Lightly flex the right leg to support the body weight. Lift the left leg to form a right angle with the trunk, flexing the knee until the foot is on a level with the right knee. Raise the left hand to nose height and the right hand to the level of the nipple. Gaze at the left middle finger. Concentrate on the *dan tian*. Repeat the movements on the opposite side.

Helps the body balance.

Ending posture (Fig. 24): Stand quietly with both hands on the navel *dan tian* for three to five minutes. Take a walk or practise a keep-fit exercise.

Note: The patient may choose one, two or three exercises from these twelve depending on the condition. It is not necessary to practise all twelve; mastering too many is not good, lest side effects occur.

Normal and Abnormal Reactions

Certain reactions, either normal or abnormal, are apt to occur during the breathing exercises. Normal reactions occur in those who adhere strictly to the requirements and experience deeply the postures, concentration, breathing and meditation. They obey all the points to be remembered. Conversely, abnormal reactions occur in those who do not follow the right way. They are usually overanxious, seeking effects blindly, and of course, disregard the directions. As a result, they fail to achieve benefits from these exercises.

Normal Reactions
The following are the reactions most commonly encountered.

1. Profuse secretion of saliva

During exercise there is an obvious increase in salivary secretion as a result of the tongue's touching the palate, which stimulates salivary secretion. Saliva thus secreted should be swallowed in several parts separately, for it is helpful to digestion. It also bears important significance in the prevention of carcinoma of the digestive system.

2. Clear-headedness and energeticness.

These usually occur during or after exercise and last for a long time. If the environment is well ventilated and the exercise lasts for over half an hour with satisfactory quietness, the exerciser will feel clear-headed, happy, relaxed and energetic and will work with higher efficiency afterward.

3. Increase of sleep

With progress in exercising the exerciser will begin to sleep more soundly and longer, overcoming fatigue and regaining energy. The effect of breathing exercises on insomnia is especially dramatic and satisfactory.

4. Sensation of warmth and mild perspiration

The body temperature of the exerciser will increase about 0.5 degree Centigrade. This commonly occurs during exercise. When concentrating on the *dan tian* or *qihai* point, the exerciser may also feel a sensation of warmth. With advancing skill the exerciser will feel warmth (internal vital energy) coursing through the *du* and *ren* channels (located along the midlines of the dorsal and ventral surfaces of the torso and head). This yields a warm and comfortable sensation.

5. Increase of gastrointestinal peristalsis and appetite

These occur after abdominal breathing exercises and may be accompanied by an increase in peristaltic sounds. These have a good effect on the digestion of food, absorption of nutrients and excretion. It is not at all strange for a skilful exerciser to experience good appetite, normal defecation, and a marked increase of body weight.

6. Itching sensation and involuntary contraction of muscles

These reactions are apt to occur and may affect the attainment of quietness. Light stroking will relieve the itching sensation. Do not scratch vigorously. For muscular contraction, just shift the attention away from the contraction and it will fade away spontaneously.

7. Vigorous metabolism

Body metabolism speeds up as the exercising progresses. Secretion of endocrine glands, salivary glands, sweat glands and sebaceous glands is greatly increased. The nails, hair and beard grow more rapidly than usual.

8. Various relaxed sensations

Feelings of relaxation other than the aforementioned ones are apt to occur. For example, the whole body may feel as if it were having a sunbath in spring.

All the above reactions are not necessarily felt by all exercisers. Some may experience more reactions, some fewer; still others may have no reactions at all. As for the time when such reactions may occur, some may be earlier, some later. Normal reactions are not the final goal of breathing exercises, hence, in principle, if they happen, make the best of it. Don't seek such reactions if they do not happen. Moreover, if they do happen, don't pay too much attention to them; otherwise you will go against the natural principles for breathing exercises.

Abnormal Reactions

1. Dizziness, headache and distention sensation in the head

The causes of these reactions are too many distracting thoughts, nervousness in fixing one's consciousness and forced meditation. In hypertension incomplete relaxation of the muscles would result in such reactions. These can be cured by the elimination of causes.

2. Chest swollen and stuffy, breathing not smooth

These are caused by excessive exercise, forced breathing and holding the breath too long, violating the principle that breathing should be natural and smooth and the principle of combination of exercise and rest. Elimination of overanxiety for success and persistence in proceeding step by step will eventually get rid of these reactions.

3. Tachycardia, pain in the chest and flank

Mainly caused by over throwing out the chest and bending the back, nervousness, holding the breath too long, counting too many numbers, etc. These problems can be avoided by complete relaxation and not paying attention to the breath until it recovers naturally.

4. Superficial breathing, abdominal distension

As a rule, these happen to exercisers who try to force their breathing to change from a thoracic type to an abdominal type, from superficial to deep. The respiratory muscles may become exhausted under such conditions. Since a deep, long and gentle breath is reached only after painstaking and persistent practice and, of course, can't be sought reluctantly, if one practises hard enough regularly, by and by one will master the main points and the breathing will become long and deep naturally.

5. Mouth and tongue dry, ears ringing, eyes blurred

These reactions often occur in those who are weak or engage in too frequent sexual activity; the heart and the kidney cannot coordinate; the *yin* and *yang* are not balanced; a weak *yang* is in the ascendant. To correct, strictly limit sexual activity. The exercises should be performed one or two days after sexual intercourse.

6. Body shakes

During exercise the head and torso or the extremities may shake or tremble and change position involuntarily. Shaking is caused by the sinking of the vital energy into the *dan tian*, which causes abnormal pressure. In such a case pulsation of the aorta with peristalsis of the digestive tract may spread over the whole body. Mild, slight and natural shaking is beneficial for overcoming fatigue. Nevertheless, the reverse effect as well as nervous symptoms will occur if one shakes consciously, vigorously and frequently. This one must avoid. Should it happen, don't exaggerate it voluntarily and it will cease by itself. There is also a breathing exercise with movement that can be performed only under the supervision and direction of an experienced physician; otherwise accidents are apt to happen.

7. Fever and chills

The cause of chills is low environmental temperature, insufficient clothing, hunger, frequent emission, severe anaemia, etc. Elimination of the cause will overcome the sensation. As for fever, it may be caused by hot weather, corpulence, eating too much meat, resulting in abundant seminal fluid, etc. Experts in breathing exercises call it overdoing it. To overcome the problems no exercise should be performed on an empty or overfull stomach. The exercise place should be well ventilated, the temperature kept at about 16 degrees C, with suitable clothing and light food. Moreover, don't get overanxious about achieving quietness. A calm mind will naturally lead to meditation.

8. Seminal emission

Generally, breathing exercises are useful for the treatment of emission. Physiologically, it is normal for emission to occur occasionally in the course of exercise. However, frequent emission results in weakness of the body and worsening of the disease. This can be overcome only by having little or no desire and by persistent exercise. Occasionally it may also be overcome by coordinating some reverse breathing exercises with contraction and elevation of the sphincter muscles.

9. Difficulty in breathing

No matter what position one selects, difficulty in breathing, restlessness, a depressed sensation in the chest and pain in the costal region are all caused by unsuitable breathing or overanxiety about one's breathing or by forced protrusion of the abdominal wall. These go against the essentials of exercise. To correct, relax and follow the principle of natural, gentle and smooth breathing. Pay more attention to exhalation than to inhalation, inhaling and exhaling through the nose or inhaling through the nose and exhaling through the mouth. That way the breathing will become natural.

10. Shortness of breath, pain and a depressed sensation in the chest

These often occur in patients suffering from pulmonary tuberculosis or emphysema and bronchiectasis who do not breathe properly. To prevent, don't get overanxious about abdominal breathing. Try to master the technique step by step. Holding the breath is prohibited for these patients.

11. Common cold

Mild common cold may occasionally occur during exercising, causing impediment of the nasal passage. Persistence in exercising will overcome it naturally. If obstruction lasts for a long time, use finger acupuncture on the *yingxiang* acupoint or simply drip ephedrine solution in the nose, However, worsening of the condition, sudden increase in body temperature, etc., require a temporary rest and drug therapy.

12. Fatigue

This often occurs if an improper posture is adopted. One's posture should not be stereotyped and copied mechanically. It should vary according to the individual. Whichever of the four posture—standing, sitting, lying or walking—one chooses, it is advisable not to exercise for too long a period.

One should start with a short period, lengthening it gradually, for beginners are not accustomed to exercising and are apt to become fatigued. They do not easily adapt to the condition.

If you feel uncomfortable, change your posture. For instance, if a supine position is not satisfactory, then lie on your side or even sit. The only requirement is "ease".

Patients with heart disease should lie on the right side, because lying on the opposite side would press the heart, causing an unpleasant sensation.

Patients with a peptic ulcer should lie on the right side to ease the transfer of food from the stomach to the intestine.

13. Lumbago and backache

Forcing the chest out will cause these. Once the position is correctly maintained, the pain will disappear naturally. Weak and aged patients should sit on a chair rather than a stool and should perform some waist movements before and after exercising. Patients of chronic nephritis should lie down, rather than sit or stand, so as to lessen the burden on the spinal column and lumbar region.

14. Distracting thoughts

Some exercisers may ordinarily have no distracting thoughts, but when they are exercising they may think of many questions and may not even be able to control their thinking. This prevents the arrival of quietude. The condition may be overcome by replacing all distracting thoughts with one thought, such as concentrating on the word *relaxation* or *quietness*. In this way most of the sensory nerve cells will be inhibited and only a few stimulated. If distracting thoughts occur frequently and are not easily controlled, just count the breaths and eventually a "unity of spirit and vital energy" will be reached.

15. Lack of calm

Some exercisers become anxious, angry and restless. In that case don't exercise reluctantly. Choose another activity, such as walking in the fresh air, drinking tea, or even taking a sedative. Resume exercising only after calmness has been restored.

16. Sensation of lightness, heaviness, pain and itching

Some exercisers may feel body lightness or heaviness, even to being unable to move immediately, pain here and there, or itching. These sensations disappear spontaneously if you aren't overanxious for quick success at the beginning, are fearless when reactions occur during exercising and are not reluctant to end the exercise.

17. Hallucination

Some people while exercising have sensations of photism and phonism—their bodies seem to get bigger or smaller. At such a time one must remain stable and not surrender one's concentration, become fearful or suspicious. Don't seek this hallucination consciously and it will disappear spontaneously after a moment.

18. Sensation of hunger

After several days' exercise hunger is apt to develop. Appropriate increase of food intake is advisable, or the therapeutic effect may be affected. Nevertheless, too much food must be avoided.

19. Diarrhoea, distention of the abdomen and abdominal ache

These may be caused by temperature changes or cold in the abdomen or by taking too much or unclean food and drink. Treatment should be applied to the cause, with drug therapy when necessary.

20. Sudden fright

During a long exercise session the exerciser may be disturbed by some external factor, such as a noise. Interrupting the exercise temporarily until one's feelings are stable will correct the abnormal reaction.

These abnormal reactions do not necessarily occur in all exercisers. Once one happens, it can be cured by the method described. To avoid undesirable reactions beginners should perform the exercises strictly under the guidance of experienced experts. They should have a good grasp and thorough understanding of some of the key links (relaxation, concentration, meditation, breathing practice) and eventually master them so as to proceed smoothly and get satisfactory therapeutic results.

Chapter II

Traditional Gymnastics for Health (Martial Arts)

Taijiquan (Shadow Boxing)

(1) Brief History

A time-honoured physical exercise, *taijiquan* has spread widely, establishing different schools. In ancient China it was a type of keep-fit martial art.

As for the origin of *taijiquan* there are conflicting reports, including records from the Tang, Song and Ming dynasties by Xu Xuanping, Zhang Sanfeng and Zhang Sanfeng (different characters in Chinese) respectively. Historical materials vary, some too brief, some legendary and unreliable. Qing Dynasty materials are not detailed enough. Most historians believe *taijiquan* was invented at the end of the Ming Dynasty by Chen Yuting.

A native of Chenjiagou, Wen County, Henan Province, Chen Yuting was a general in the late Ming Dynasty. Unwilling to serve the Qing Dynasty after the overthrow of the Ming Dynasty, he lived in seclusion in his native village and devoted his life to martial arts. Starting with the famous general Qi Jiguang's *Martial Arts Classic of 32 Postures*, Chen Yuting proposed 5 sets of *taijiquan*, a set of 108 long martial-arts postures and a set of *pao chui* martial arts.

Chen's *Taijiquan* shadow boxing has been passed down from generation to generation until today. Hence, it is called Chen's *taijiquan*. Later Yang Lu-chan of Yongnian, Hebei Province, modified Chen's *taijiquan* to form a new set without jumping, with even and smooth velocity and extensions. The latter was further improved by Yang's son, Yang Jianhou, and grandson, Yang Chengfu. Hence the name Yang's *taijiquan* which has considerable popularity because of its remarkable therapeutic efficacy and rehabilitative action.

Later, other schools of *taijiquan* appeared. Two developed by the men named Wu and Sun became as famous and popular as Yang's.

Basically, all *taijiquan* postures evolved from Chen's *taijiquan* and bear a successive relation. Though the styles vary in complexity and pattern, the principle of combining soft with hard, with soft predominant, is primarily the same.

Since the founding of New China the old gymnastic art has been receiving special attention developing into a favourite exercise for many people.

In fact, *taijiquan* combines exercise of body, mind and vital energy. In exercising the body, it relaxes all the body muscles, with gentle, slow and smooth movements that go from simple to complex, from easy to difficult, varied according to the individual. In exercising the mind, it focuses the attention, free from distracting thoughts, so as to rest the cerebral cortex and achieve psychosomatic health. As for one's vital energy, *taijiquan* deepens the breathing to an abdominal type. Since *taijiquan* is a traditional martial-arts exercise, its exercise of the mind, body and vital energy should be viewed as an exercise in martial technique and thus adapted to one's own condition in its application as rehabilitative medicine.

(2) Effects
(a) On the central nervous system

In practising *taijiquan* one must concentrate the mind, free it of distractions, seeking tranquillity while moving and applying consciousness rather than applying force. All these act favourably on the activity of the cerebrum. The movements in *taijiquan* must be integrated throughout in a continuous process, moving the whole body when it moves. These complex movements can be accomplished only under the direction of the brain, which, in turn affects the central nervous system.

(b) On the circulatory and respiratory systems

Essentially *taijiquan* exercises, internally, the vital energy and, externally, the muscles, bones and skin. Respiration should be deep, long, natural and gentle, concentrated on the *dan tian* point an even and regular respiration that combines movement of the diaphragm and abdominal muscles. Such movement improves blood circulation, dilates the coronary arteries, strengthens oxidation and reduction reactions. All the changes strengthen the cardiac muscles and lay a foundation for preventing heart diseases.

(c) On the digestive system

Since *taijiquan* uses an abdominal type of respiration, it stimulates the digestive tract in a mechanical way to promote its circulation and increase secretion and is therefore good for curing diseases caused by disturbance of the sympathetic nervous system, such as peptic ulcer, gastroptosis and dyspepsia.

(3) Essentials of Practice
(a) Natural and relaxed

A quiet, tranquil mind is required throughout the whole process. Relaxation and tranquillity should be mastered to calm the cerebral cortex and subcerebral centres. The muscles, joints and viscera should be relaxed as well. The head, shoulders, waist, hips, the whole body are all relaxed and comfortable.

(b) Correct posture

During practice the trunk should be straight, the apex of the head in line with the crotch. The following postures should be avoided: thrusting out the chest, protruding the abdomen, lowering the head, bending the waist or arms, protruding the buttocks. The chin is retracted a little, and the tip of the tongue touches the hard palate. The mouth is shut and smiling.

(c) Harmonious movements

All the movements should be directed by the mind and should be smooth and rounded. It is necessary to accomplish a harmonious, even, continuous movement, with relative stability of the joints and muscles. The movements are rounded without sharpness or interruption, and should be performed with the waist serving as axis for the extremities. The neck turns smoothly, following the eyes. Weighted and weightless steps should be strictly differentiated. Before taking a step, be sure the body weight is securely on one leg, then move another leg slowly. Only in this way can you keep your balance.

(d) Sinking of vital energy to the *dan tian*

Breathing should be natural (after mastering the movements, you may adopt abdominal breathing). Air should flow through the nostrils in natural abdominal breathing. As the whole body relaxes, the lower abdomen should feel substantial and the chest easy. Movements of the diaphragm and waist massage the viscera.

(4) Movements

Originally *taijiquan* movements were difficult and complex. For instance, high jumps were part of Chen's *taijiquan*. Later modifications suited *taijiquan* for health care. After Liberation, in order to popularize *taijiquan*, the State Physical Culture and Sports Commission, formulated a simplified *taijiquan* of twenty-four or forty-eight movements. Some patients, however, can't support even simplified *taijiquan* and must practise a single movement or a few individual movements, depending on the illness, physical condition, age, etc. In any event, perseverance is of utmost importance. The nature and complexity of the movements may be increased gradually until a whole series of movements from any school can be tolerated.

Here a few exercises are introduced ranging from easy to complex.

(a) *Taiji* movements

1. To relax the whole body, practise a breathing exercise first, then the *taiji* exercise. Those who are severely ill and weak may go directly into the *taiji* exercise. For the breathing exercise the knees are slightly bent and the arms are rounded in front of the chest.

2. Natural breathing: The breathing muscles are also

relaxed as the whole body relaxes. Respiration, whether through the mouth or the nose, is natural.

3. The eyes may or may not be shut. Concentrate a bit on the *dan tian* point to get rid of distracting thoughts.

4. Once relaxed, you can begin the movements. During the whole exercise the knees should be slightly flexed as for the breathing exercises. Let yourself move freely. If you feel like moving quickly, move quickly; slowly, move slowly; make large movements or small movements. After a while the movements will become automatic. Let this happen naturally. Don't be afraid of it or try to force it.

5. Stop gradually when you want to end the exercise. After finishing the movements, open your eyes and take a slow walk for several minutes. Do some deep breathing or massage the face or scalp.

Taiji movements are basically the same as *taijiquan* itself, except they are completely free. Thus anyone can practise without difficulty.

(b) Selection of *taijiquan* exercises

Any of the following *taiji* movements can be selected if a complete series of movements cannot be undertaken.

(5) Selected *Taijiquan* Movements
Section One
Beginning Movements
(1) Stand erect naturally with the feet, shoulder width apart, the arms hanging naturally, eyes gazing forward (Fig. 25). Don't intentionally protrude the chest or pull in the stomach.

Points to remember: head and neck erect, chin retracted, chest relaxed. Moves should be natural and the mind concentrated.

(2) Raise arms slowly upward and forward to shoulder height, palms facing downward (Figs. 26 and 27). Lower arms, bending knees slightly at same time (Fig. 28).

Parting the Wild Horse's Mane

Continuing from the above posture, turn slightly to the right and shift weight to the right leg. Draw left foot beside the right one. Raise right hand to right side of chest with forearm horizontal, palm downward; move left hand in an arc under right one, palm upward, as if holding a ball with left toe touching ground. Gaze at the right hand (Figs. 29-30). Step forward and left with the left leg bowed, while the right straight. At the same time move the left hand out and up, the right hand down and back. The left fingers point upward at eyebrow height. The right hand is alongside the right hip, palm down. Gaze forward (Figs. 31-32).

Points to remember: The trunk should be straight. Hands should move in an arc. The chest should be relaxed. Trunk should turn with the waist as axis, and foot and hand movements should be gradual, even and natural. The same movements are performed on the right side.

The White Crane Spreads Its Wings

Continuing from the above posture, turn upper body slightly to the left. Move right arm, palm upward, in an arc to form a holding-ball gesture (Fig. 33).

Draw right foot half a step towards left foot, then sit back a little, shifting weight to right leg. Move left leg forward a little with toes touching ground. Separate hands obliquely towards upper right and lower left

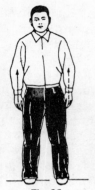

Fig. 25

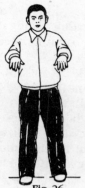

Fig. 26

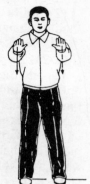

Fig. 27

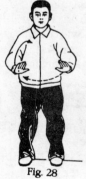

Fig. 28

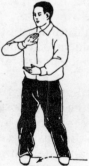

Fig. 29

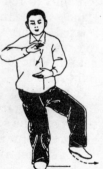

Fig. 30

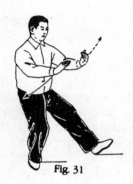

Fig. 31

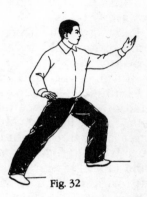

Fig. 32

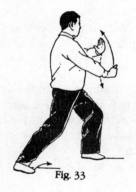

Fig. 33

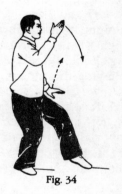

Fig. 34

57

respectively. Raise right hand to head height on right with palm facing in. Drop left hand down in front of left hip with palm facing down, fingers forward. Gaze forward (Fig. 34).

Points to remember: Don't thrust the chest out. Arms form a semicircle. Left knee bends slightly.

Section Two
Brushing Knee and Twisting Step

Continuing from the above posture, drop the right hand downward, then move it upward in an arc with palm facing upward. Move left hand in an arc from lower left to upper right until it reaches the right chest. Turn trunk to right at same time. Gaze at palm of right hand (Figs. 35 and 36). Turn trunk left, step left leg left forward obliquely with knee bent over toe to form a bow step. Move right arm back past right ear then push forward, palm out, fingers pointing up; sweep left hand down to brush left knee and return to hip, palm down, fingers forward. Gaze at fingers of right hand (Figs. 37 and 38).

Points to remember: Trunk should be stable and upright. Do not protrude buttocks. Shoulders and elbows should be relaxed.

Playing the Lute

Draw right leg near left heel and put weight on right leg. Lift left toe and bend knee slightly. At same time raise left hand to nose level with elbow slightly flexed. Draw right hand back to inside of left elbow. Gaze at left index finger (Figs. 39 and 40).

Point to remember: Left hand should move in an arc.

Stepping Back with Rolling Arms

Continuing from the above posture, draw the right

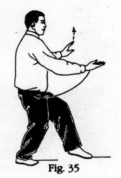

Fig. 35

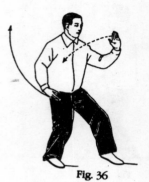

Fig. 36

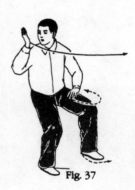

Fig. 37

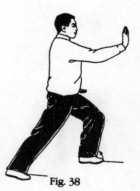

Fig. 38

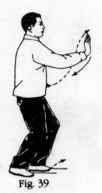

Fig. 39

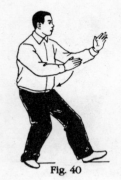

Fig. 40

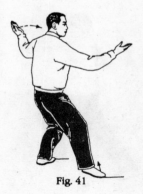

Fig. 41

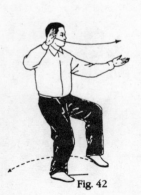

Fig. 42

hand back, turning the palm up and passing the lower abdomen, then draw an arc upward. (Fig. 41). Turn the left palm up and gaze at the left hand (Fig. 42). Bend the right arm past the right ear, then push it forward, palm out (Fig. 43). Draw the left arm back past the left rib, lift the left leg gently and step back. Draw an arc upward with the left hand. Gaze at the right hand with palm upward. (Fig. 44).

Points to remember: When stepping back, the toes should touch the ground first. The left leg steps back obliquely towards the left, the right leg obliquely towards the right. The knees remain bent. Steps back should be poised and stable. The eyes should first follow the trunk to turn left or right, then transfer the gaze to the hand in front. Movements on the left and right sides are exactly the same.

Section Three

Grasping the Peacock's Tail (left)

This exercise may be done independently or as a continuation of the previous one.

Turn the trunk to the right. Move the left hand from lower left to upper right in an arc and stop at the right side of the waist. Flex the right elbow and raise the right arm to chest level to form a holding-ball gesture. At the same time point the right toe out, and draw the left leg near the right leg, with left toe touching the ground (Figs. 45 and 46). Step the left foot left with the right toe turning inward as you move the left arm towards the left shoulder, bending it like a bow and pushing it forward horizontally with palm facing inward. Drop the right hand down to the right hip, palm down. Gaze at the left forearms (Fig 47).

Turn the trunk slightly left, push the left hand

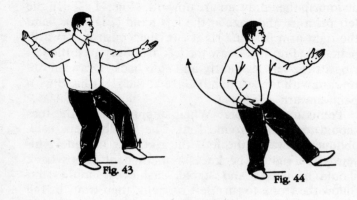

Fig. 43   Fig. 44

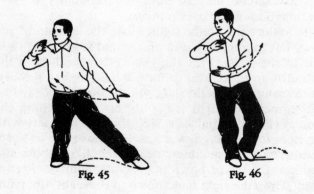

Fig. 45   Fig. 46

forward with palm turning downward, and raise right arm with palm turning upward, passing before the abdomen up to the lower of the left forearm. Draw both hands back to the right in an arc (with right palm downward, left upward, as if grasping and stroking a peacock's tail), passing in front of the abdomen until the right arm extends sideways at shoulder's height, the left arm bent horizontally in front of the right part of the chest, palm facing back. Shift weight on the right leg; gaze at right hand.

Turn the trunk slightly left, bend the right arm back with palm outward to the inside of the left wrist (about five centimetres apart) (Fig. 48). Separate the two hands, both palms facing downward at shoulder height. Bend right leg, sit backward, shifting weight on the right leg and lift left toe. At the same time bend hands to the front of abdomen, fingers forward, palms downward. Shift weight forward, push palms forward and upward; bend left leg forward to form a bow step. Gaze forward (Fig. 49).

Grasping the Peacock's Tail (right)

Starting from the end of the previous movement, shift the weight back onto the right leg. Point the left toe inward. Move the right hand to the right in an arc, then move it from right to left, passing in front of the abdomen, and stop at the left side of the waist with palm facing upward. Flex the left hand in front of the chest to form a holding-ball gesture with the right one. The weight then moves onto the left leg. Move the right leg near the left one with the toes touching the ground. Step towards the right in a bow step. At the same time move the right arm to the right and flex like a bow. Drop the left hand to the left hip, palm facing downward (Figs. 50 and 51). Follow Figures 52 through 55 to complete the exercise. Left side and right side are exactly the same, simply reversed.

Section Four

Single Whip (Figs. 56-60)

The exercise may be continued from the above posture or performed independently. Move the left leg leftward a step and a half, "sit" back and shift the weight onto it. Turn the right toe in a little. Turn the trunk to the left. Move both arms, the left above, the right below, towards the left by passing before the chest until the left arm is sideways at shoulder level and the right arm is in front of the left subcostal region. Gaze at the left hand. Shift body weight gradually to the right leg. Move left leg next to right leg. Move right hand towards upper back until it reaches shoulder level. Hook right hand. Drop left hand down and move rightward in an arc, passing the abdomen, towards right shoulder, with palm facing inward. Gaze at left hand. Turn trunk slightly towards left back. Step on left leg in a bow step. Turn left palm at wrist and push it forward, palm facing out and fingers at eye level. Flex both arms a little. Gaze at left hand.

Points to remember: Keep trunk erect and waist relaxed. In the end, right elbow should be bent slightly and left elbow directly above left knee. Drop both shoulders. All transitional movements should be well coordinated and harmonious.

Cloud Hands (Figs. 61 and 62):

Stand erect. Step sideways to the left. Shift weight to right leg and turn trunk gradually towards right with left toe pointing inward. Move the left hand in an arc passing before abdomen towards upper right until it

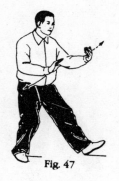

Fig. 47

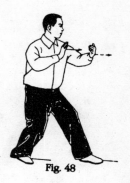

Fig. 48

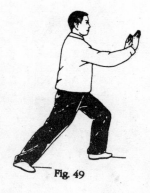

Fig. 49

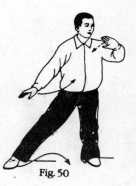

Fig. 50

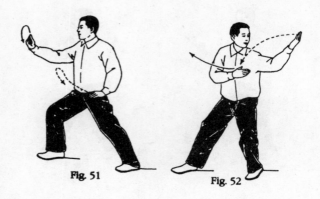

Fig. 51 Fig. 52

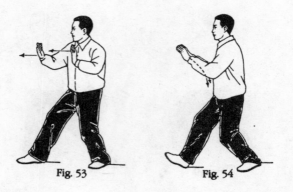

Fig. 53 Fig. 54

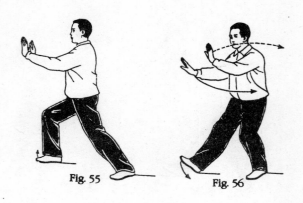

Fig. 55

Fig. 56

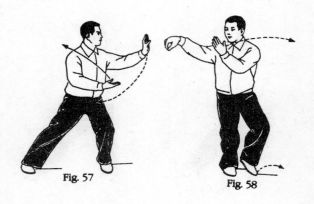

Fig. 57

Fig. 58

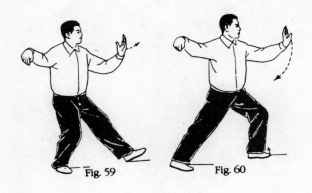

Fig. 59

Fig. 60

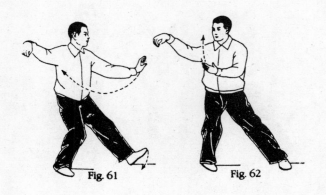

Fig. 61

Fig. 62

reaches right shoulder level, with palm facing backward obliquely. Gaze at left hand. Shift weight gradually to the left. Move left hand from the right by passing in front of the head, palm facing inward, towards the left, turning at the waist. Right hand moves from lower right towards upper left by passing before the abdomen until it reaches the left shoulder, with palm facing backward obliquely. Meanwhile, move right foot towards the left until they are ten to twenty centimetres apart. Gaze at right hand. Then move right hand towards right side and move left hand in an arc towards right shoulder by passing before the abdomen, with palm facing backward obliquely. Turn right palm towards right side. Step sideways on left leg. Gaze at left hand.

Points to remember: Waist serves as axis in turning trunk. Avoid up or down movements of the trunk. Muscles are all relaxed. Arms turn and move with the waist in a natural, smooth way. The body weight should be stable when moving lower extremities. Eyes follow hand movements.

Section Five

Reaching High on the Horse (Figs. 63 and 64)

Continuing from the previous posture, move the right heel half step forward. Both hands turn palms upward. Bend the elbows slightly. Meanwhile, turn the trunk slightly towards the right and raise the left heel. Gaze at the left hand. Push the right hand forward past the right ear. Draw the left hand back to the left loin with the palm facing upward. Gaze at the right hand.

Points to remember: Trunk is upright, no bending of the trunk and chest when pushing the right hand; it should be eyebrow height with the weight falling on the

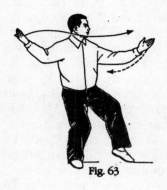

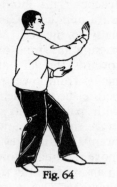

Fig. 63　　　　　　　　　　　　Fig. 64

right leg.

Kicking with Right Heel (Figs. 65-68)

Continuing from the above posture, move the left hand forward with palm upward until it crosses the right wrist with palm downward. Separate the arms with the palms pointing downward obliquely. Meanwhile the left leg takes a bow step. Shift body weight to it, while the right leg stretches straight naturally. The hands turn first outward, then inward in arc until they cross in front of the chest, both palms facing inward, the right hand in front of the left. At the same time move the right foot towards the left with toes touching the ground. Gaze between the hands. Then draw the arms sideways in arc horizontally, with palms facing out. Bend right knee and lift right foot, kicking slowly forward with the right heel. Gaze at the right hand. Clench the fists loosely and keep the arms in an arc with shoulders and elbows fully relaxed.

Double Peaks Pierce Ears

Raise right knee and bring left hand back, up then

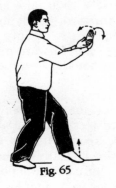

Fig. 65

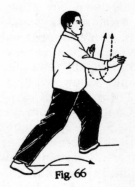

Fig. 66

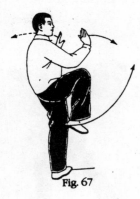

Fig. 67

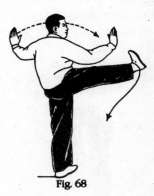

Fig. 68

forward in arc. With both palms up, lower hands in arc
to each side of right knee, gaze forward (Fig. 69). Drop
hands down, clenching fists loosely, then raise arms in
arc from sideways and thrust forward, hands in loose
fists, palm towards palm about ten to twenty centimetres apart, at ear level, as you step forward on right
foot and shift weight on it. Shoulders and elbows
should be lowered (Fig. 70).

Turning and Kicking with Left Heel

Continuing from previous position, relax waist and
hips. Squat over right leg with toes pointing slightly
outward. Turn trunk leftward. Relax fists and extend
fingers. Raise both hands upward laterally to shoulder
height in arc, palms facing out. Gaze at left hand. Shift
weight onto right leg; draw left leg near right leg. Draw
both hands from lateral towards medial in arc to cross
in front of chest, with the left wrist outside the right
one. Palms face in. Gaze forward (Figs. 71 and 72).
Kick with left heel and stretch arms out sideways. Gaze
at left hand (Fig. 73).

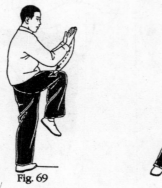

Fig. 69

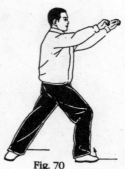

Fig. 70

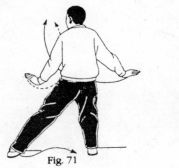

Fig. 71

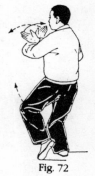

Fig. 72

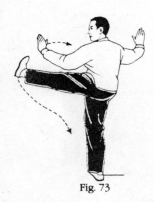

Fig. 73

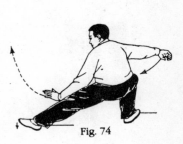

Fig. 74

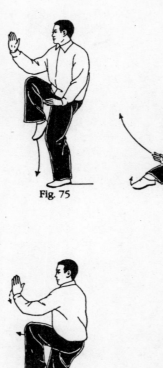

Fig. 75

Fig. 76

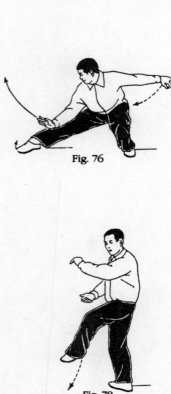

Fig. 77

Fig. 78

Section Six

Low Single Stand (left side)

Continuing from previous position, stand erect with left toe touching ground, body weight on right leg. Right palm is hooked. Move left hand rightward until it reaches right armpit. Gaze at left hand. Squat slowly on right leg and move left leg leftward as if to spring and jump. Move left hand downward and leftward, passing inside of left thigh. Gaze at left hand (Fig. 74). Shift body weight gradually onto left leg until it is wholly transferred to left. Lift right heel, then right knee upward and forward. Move right hand forward until it reaches right hip. Then stand steady on left leg and gradually stand up straight, but with knee slightly bent. Meanwhile raise bent right knee to navel height with toes pointing forward and foot dropped naturally. Turn right palm out and raise right hand until tips of fingers reach eyebrow height, palm facing leftward. Drop elbow towards knee, holding about a fist width apart. Left palm presses down; right palm points upward. Gaze forward. Stand steady on one foot (Fig. 75).

Low Single Stand (right side)

Movements are reverse of previous posture. Touch ground with right toe, body weight on left leg. Turn body to left, with left toe as its axis and heel pointing slightly inward. Meanwhile raise left hand backward and form a hooked hand. Draw right palm leftward in arc until it reaches left armpit. Gaze at right hand. Continue as for left side. Standing knee should be slightly bent and well balanced (Figs. 76-77).

Section Seven

Shuttle (right and left)

Stand erect. Extend left leg with torso turned slightly leftward, then drop left foot onto ground with toes pointing outward. Raise right heel to form a half "seated cross-legged." Hands form ball-holding gesture in front of chest. Move right foot near left foot, with left toes touching ground. Gaze at left forearm. Step forward on right leg to form a right bow step. Meanwhile pass right hand in front of face, turn palm and stop at right temple, palm facing upward obliquely. Then push left hand out in front of trunk, with palm facing forward. Gaze at left hand (Figs. 80-82). Shift body weight backward a little to move right toe out a little. Then shift weight to right leg. Left foot follows immediately stopping close to the inside of right foot, right toe touching ground. Both hands are in front of right side of chest as if holding a balloon (right hand in upper position). Gaze at right forearm. Move left leg half a step so left leg forms bow; straddles right leg straight. Raise left arm to ear height. Right palm passes in front of left chest to point upward and outward just below left forearm. Gaze in left forward direction (Figs. 83-84).

Needle on the Sea Bottom (Figs. 86 and 87)

Stand with legs shoulder width apart. Turn torso leftward. Take one step with left leg, followed by half a step with right leg. Shift weight to right leg. Then move left leg forward a little, toes touching ground. Meanwhile draw right hand back across torso until it reaches right ear. Immediately thrust right hand downward palm facing left, fingers downward obliquely; while left hand moves down in arc to left hip, palm downward, fingers forward. Gaze forward.

Points to remember: Trunk shouldn't bow down too

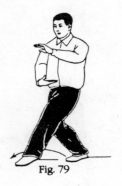

Fig. 79

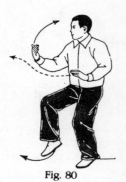

Fig. 80

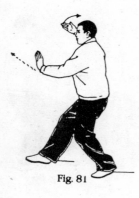

Fig. 81

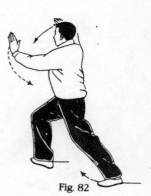

Fig. 82

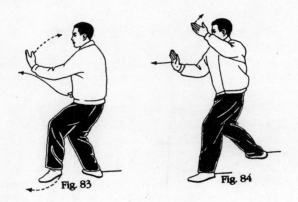

Fig. 83

Fig. 84

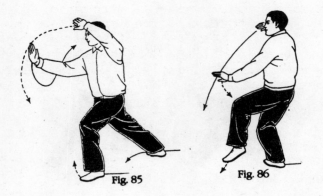

Fig. 85

Fig. 86

much. Avoid dropping head and protruding buttocks. While thrusting right hand, shoulder shouldn't incline. Left leg is slightly bent.

Opening the Arms (Figs. 88-90)

Turn torso a little to right. Step out on left leg to form a bow. Pass right arm in front of trunk and flex it above head, with palm facing obliquely outward and thumb downward. Push left hand forward at same time, passing in front of the chest with palm facing forward and thumb upward. Gaze at left hand.

Revolving, Blocking and Punching (Figs. 91-94)

Bend right leg and shift body weight onto it. Point left toe in and turn trunk to the right backward. Then shift weight to left leg. Meanwhile right hand moves with revolving trunk, rightward and downward clenching fist, passing in front of abdomen and stopping at left costal region, the palm facing downward in a fist. Raise left palm and stop at upper portion in front of head, the arm forming a semicircle, the palm facing upward obliquely. Gaze forward, then turn trunk to the right and turn right fist facing upward when passing chest thrusting forward, palm up, and drop left hand down beside left hip. Draw right foot back and without touching the ground step forward immediately pointing toe out. Gaze at right fist with palm inward; push left hand forward, draw right fist back to right hip. Step forward on left leg in bow step as right fist thrusts forward, left arm bends back. Gaze at right fist.

As If Obstructing (Figs. 95-97)

Continuing from the above, extend the left hand around and under the right wrist with the right fist opened to a flat palm. Draw both palms, facing ·upward, back slowly. "Sit" back a little on right leg,

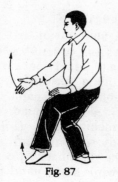

Fig. 87

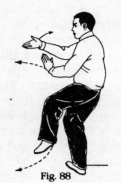

Fig. 88

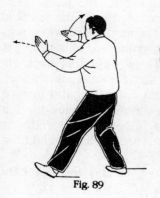

Fig. 89

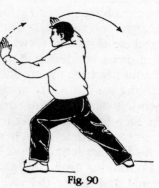

Fig. 90

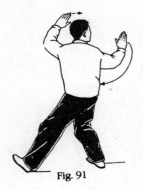

Fig. 91

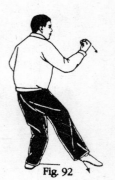

Fig. 92

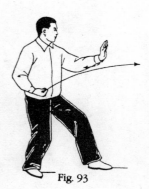

Fig. 93

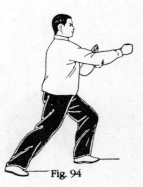

Fig. 94

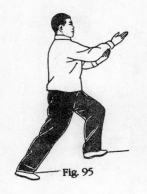

Fig. 95

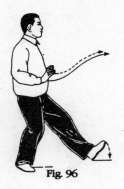

Fig. 96

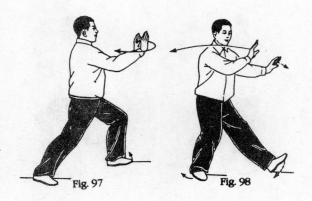

Fig. 97   Fig. 98

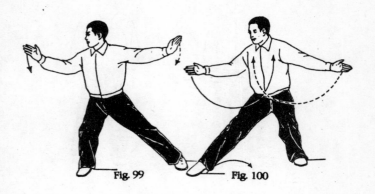

Fig. 99   Fig. 100

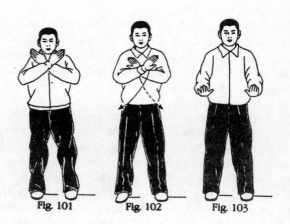

Fig. 101   Fig. 102   Fig. 103

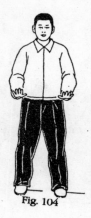

Fig. 104

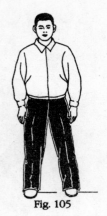

Fig. 105

pointing left toe upward. Gaze forward. Draw both hands towards chest, turn palms to face forward and push forward simultaneously. Take a left bow step. Gaze between the two palms.

Points to remember: When "sitting" back, don't bend back upward. Buttocks shouldn't protrude. As arms are drawn back, following backward movement of the trunk, elbows should move out a little. Do not draw straight back.

Crossed Hands (Figs. 98-101)

Continuing from the above position, shift body weight to right leg; point left toe in. Turn body to the right, with right hand following trunk around on the horizontal. Thus both left and right arms extend sideways with elbows dropped naturally. Right toe moves with the body, pointing out to form a right bow step. Gaze at right hand. Shift weight slowly towards left leg. Move right leg leftward one step. At same time move both arms down, then up, crossing in front of the trunk to form crossed hands with palms facing inward, the right arm outside. Gaze forward.

Ending (Figs. 102-105)

Continuing from the above, turn both palms down and move beside hips. Gaze forward.

Points to remember: separate hands before lowering. Gaze straight ahead.

2. *Yijinjing* (Muscle-Transforming Classic)

The *Yijinjing* is an ancient set of exercises for relaxing and extending muscles and tendons and reinforcing body strength. In ancient China writings by a wise man were called "Classic." That a series of gymnastic exercises were so ranked denotes how highly people thought of these exercises.

The exercises are as follows:

1. Presenting Pestle (1) by Wei Tuo (Fig. 106)

Stand erect with feet about shoulder width apart. Raise both arms, as if holding a balloon, to chest level with fingers of two hands touching. Incline head forward a little, concentrating on tip of nose. The mind is easy and relaxed, the breath natural. Stand quietly for five minutes.

2. Presenting Pestle (2) by Wei Tuo (Fig. 107)

Continuing from previous posture, bring feet together. Extend arms sideways at shoulder height with palms facing downward. The eyes see nothing. The ears hear nothing. The mind is free from any distracting thoughts and calm.

3. Presenting Pestle (3) by Wei Tuo (Fig. 108)

Continuing from previous posture, raise arms as if

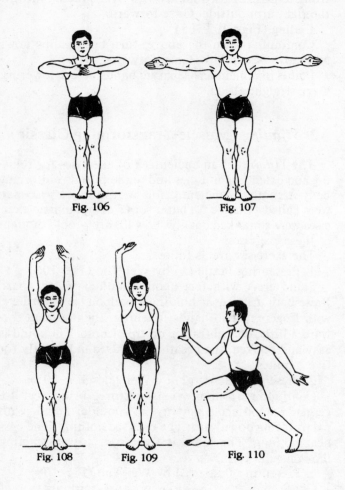

Fig. 106

Fig. 107

Fig. 108

Fig. 109

Fig. 110

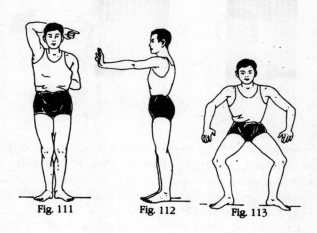

Fig. 111   Fig. 112   Fig. 113

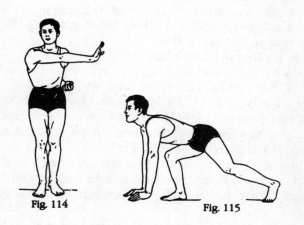

Fig. 114   Fig. 115

87

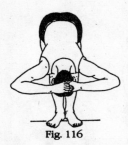

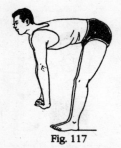

Fig. 116   Fig. 117

supporting the sky, with palms facing upward. Stand on tiptoe. Gaze upward. Shut mouth and bite teeth with tongue's tip touching the hard palate. Breathe through the nose. Adjust the breath and rest the mind.

4. Picking Stars (Fig. 109)

Continuing from previous posture, stand with heels dropping down. Drop one hand down behind the waist with the other still over the head. Gaze at upper hand. Inhale through nose and exhale through mouth. Repeat movements on other side.

5. Pulling the Cow's Tail. (Fig. 110)

Move right arm and leg forward, left arm and leg back. Right hand should be level with head and right leg slightly flexed. Left leg presses down slightly. Direct vital energy to the *dan tian*. Contract arm muscles. Gaze at the fist. Repeat movements on opposite side.

6. Holding Sabre (Fig. 111)

Stand erect. Turn head to left and bend left arm around back. Bend right arm behind and hand around head. Tense muscles. Repeat movement on opposite side.

7. Extending Claws and Showing Wings (Fig. 112)

Stand erect and stare sideways angrily. Push hands

forward, then draw back. Do seven times.

8. Dropping Three Plates (Fig. 113)

Touch hard palate with tongue. Open eyes and close mouth. Feet are apart and body squatting. Press palms downward as if clawing something, then turn palms up and stand up straight. Both feet remain on the same place. Do seven times.

9. Blue Dragon Stretches Its Claws (Fig. 114)

Stand erect, turn obliquely to the left. Stretch right arm, passing in front of forehead. Stretch fingers. Draw left arm back to left subcostal region. Clench fist. Contract shoulder and back muscles. Gaze forward. Remain calm. Repeat movements on opposite side.

10. The Hungry Tiger Springs for Preys (Fig. 115)

Support body on all fours, feet separated, forward and back. Extend head up and back as far as possible. Keep back horizontal. Breathe through nose smoothly and evenly.

11. Arching the Back (Fig. 116)

Stand up. Clasp head with hands. Bend low so head drops under perineum. Close mouth, bite with teeth and touch tip of tongue to hard palate. Bow down forcefully. The ears hear nothing.

12. Wagging the Tail (Fig. 117)

Both feet are straight; both arms forcefully touch the ground. Open eyes wide and raise head. Concentrate easily. Stand on tiptoe, then raise and stamp on heels forcefully twenty-one times. Raise either sideways sit arms to horizontal level seven times each. Afterwards sit cross-legged. Gently close eyes and mouth. Breathe through nose. Calmly adjust breath. Sit quietly.

Five-Animal Exercises

In the second century A.D. a famous physician, Hua Tuo (?-208), took traditional exercises imitating the movements of birds and beasts as the basis for a series of gymnastic exercises called Five-Animal Exercises.

Essentials of Practice

(1) Muscles should be relaxed. Head is erect, shoulders and elbows dropped and relaxed, chest relaxed. Avoid protrusion of abdomen and buttocks. Waist and hips are relaxed. The whole body is natural and easy, the face smiling. In other words, only with complete relaxation can the movements be performed so that soft exists within hard and hard exists within soft. Then spiritual comfort and complete ease can be reached after practice.

(2) In concentrating on the *dan tian* focus the mind only lightly on the navel; don't exaggerate the focusing or nervous tension will result, leading to undesirable reactions.

(3) Breathe deeply several times before exercising to help establish abdominal breathing in which the abdomen protrudes slightly in inhalation and retracts a little in exhalation. This will help achieve a light upper body and solid lower body. In middle-aged and old people it is apt to develop a heavy head and light feet, or strength in the upper body and weakness in the lower. The movements can be active and free only when the lower part of the body is stable and strong. This is what is called standing like a pine and sitting like a bell.

(4) In both form and spirit the movements should

resemble the animal being imitated and should be natural and free.

To be more specific, in practising the tiger exercise one should look fierce, with flashing eyes, springing movements, fighting postures, etc.; for the deer, movements include stretching the body, running, turning the head and extending the neck; for the monkey,picking peaches and climbing trees; for the bear, sluggish movements and squatting; for the crane, spreading the wings, flying, gliding, standing on one foot, etc.

A weak person may omit the more difficult movements.

Tiger (Figs. 118-120)

Left side: Stand erect. Step forward on left foot so that feet are one foot apart with left knee flexed. Move right arm from back to front over the head, then forward, hand forming a tiger's claw. Flex wrist at head level with palm facing downward. Left arm is behind with palm facing upward. Shake left arm forcefully twice as right arm, making use of this force, stretches forward and back twice.

Movements on right side are the reverse of left side.

Deer (Figs. 121-123)

Left side: Stand erect. Step forward on left foot so that feet are a foot apart; weight is on right leg as torso inclines backward. Raise right arm so that middle finger is at head level, palm about a fist's width from the nose. Gaze at palm. Left arm is behind, a fist's width from waist with palm facing backward. Thrust chest out naturally and look up. Reverse hands and feet and repeat movements on right side.

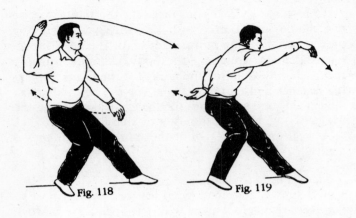

Fig. 118   Fig. 119

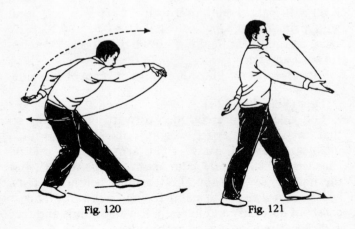

Fig. 120   Fig. 121

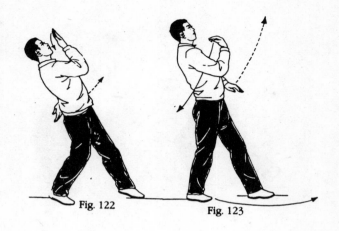

Fig. 122

Fig. 123

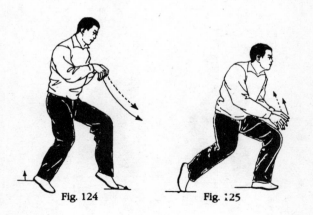

Fig. 124

Fig. 125

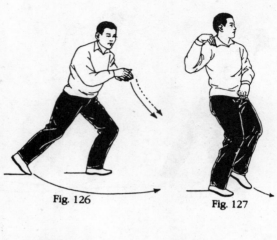

Fig. 126   Fig. 127

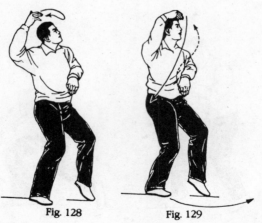

Fig. 128   Fig. 129

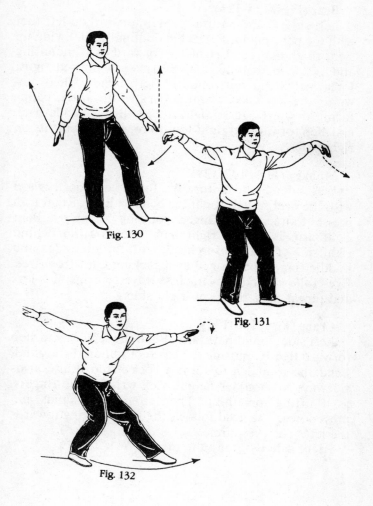

Fig. 130

Fig. 131

Fig. 132

Bear (Figs. 124-126)

Left side: Stand naturally. Step forward on left foot with toe pointing in. Retract abdominal wall. Swing up right thigh and bend right leg forward as if mounting and riding sidesaddle. Upper arms are pressed tight; forearms extend horizontally. Both hands "float" towards the left knee, about a fist's width apart, palms facing down. Gaze straight ahead. Bring hands back and step forward on right foot to repeat movements on right side.

Monkey (Figs. 127-129)

Left side: Stand naturally. Touch left toe forward with the heel raised. Right leg bends a little. Right arm presses thoracic wall, fingers pointing downward. Bent right arm is raised; right hand moves from behind right side of head to forehead, with thumb, index and middle fingers positioned as if picking fruit from tree. Eyes follow hand movements. Reverse arms and legs and repeat movements on right side.

Crane (Figs. 130-132)

Left side: Stand naturally. Bend the left leg and step forward lightly, putting the left foot flat on the ground. Bend the right leg to form a cock's step. Raise arms sideways to shoulder height, flex wrists, drop fingers, as if lifting something. Then stretch out hands and press down. The head follows the leg, swinging towards the left. The eyes circle.

Right side is simply the reverse of left.

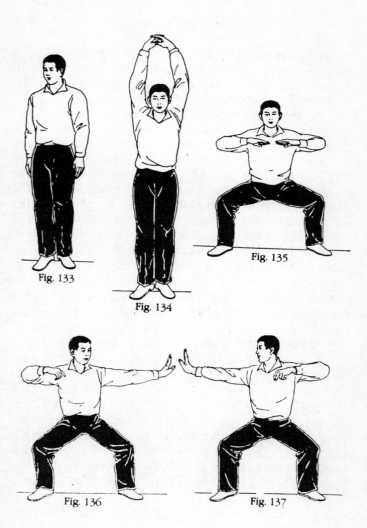

Fig. 133

Fig. 134

Fig. 135

Fig. 136

Fig. 137

Eight-Part Exercise

This set of simple, easily mastered folk exercises has long been popular and produced satisfactory results. In Chinese the exercise is called Eight Bolts of Silk, denoting it is as precious as silk.

1. Supporting the Sky with the Arms

Stand erect with feet shoulder width apart; gaze forward (Fig. 133). Muscles are all relaxed, head erect, shoulders dropped, waist and hips relaxed. Stretch fingers; dig toes into ground. Smile. Breathe through the nose. After three to five minutes of standing quietly, concentrate on the navel to achieve a state of upper lightness and lower solidity for the cultivation of vital energy. Raise both arms sideways gently until hands are over head. Intertwine fingers and turn palms upward, as if supporting the sky. Stand on toes (Fig. 134). Lower arms and heels. Repeat movements several times, coordinating breathing: inhale deeply when stretching arms upward, retracting abdominal wall. Exhale when lowering arms, abdomen protruding.

2. Shooting Arrow on Both Sides (Figs. 135-138)

Stand erect. Move left leg leftward and squat low. Cross both arms in front of chest, then flex arms horizontally, raising elbows to shoulder height. Gaze at left hand. Clench left fist, then raise left index finger upward. Next stretch left thumb to form a "V." Extend left arm towards the left until straight, turning head to gaze at left hand. Clench right fist and pull right elbow back as if shooting arrow. Recover original position. Move right foot rightward and squat low. Repeat movements for left side.

Do exercise several times. Inhale when shooting,

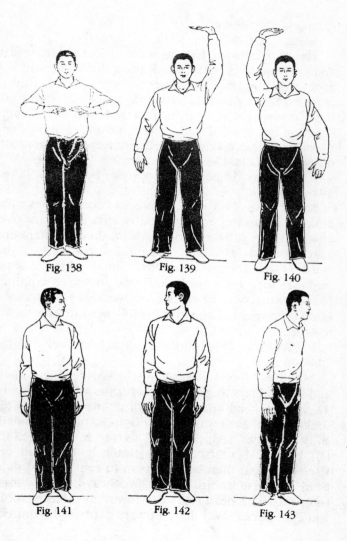

Fig. 138   Fig. 139   Fig. 140

Fig. 141   Fig. 142   Fig. 143

exhale when recovering.

3. Raising One Arm (Figs. 139 and 140)

Stand erect with feet parallel and shoulder width apart. Drop arms naturally. Raise right hand upward, arm stretching straight, palm facing upward, fingers close together, pointing leftward. Meanwhile press left hand downward with palm facing downward, fingers pointing forward. Inhale when raising arm, exhale when restoring to original position. Repeat movements on opposite side. Do several times.

4. Turning Head and Looking Backward (Figs. 141-143)

Stand erect with palms close to thighs. Keep torso still while turning head gradually leftward. Gaze over left shoulder; inhale. Return after a short moment and gaze forward, exhaling. Turn head gradually rightward. Gaze over right shoulder; inhale. After a short moment turn head back and gaze forward, exhaling. Do several times. To amplify movement turn torso at same time; gaze at opposite heel. Other movements are identical.

5. Shaking Head and Swaying Buttocks (Figs. 144-146)

Move left foot sideward in wide stride. Bend knees and squat. Press thighs with palms, thumbs pointing in. Then sway head and torso towards the left with head shaking left downward as far as possible. Meanwhile sway buttocks right, upward as far as possible, the left buttock bent first, then stretched, the right one stretched first, then bent. Return to centre, then sway head and torso towards left again. Sway head and torso rightward with head right, downward as far as possible, while buttocks sway left, upward with right buttock

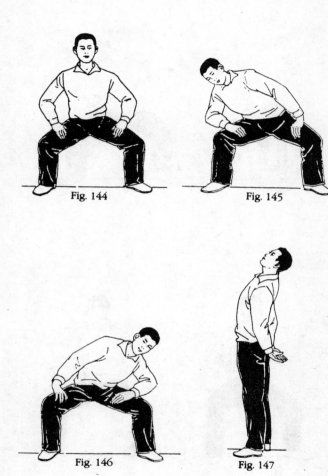

Fig. 144

Fig. 145

Fig. 146

Fig. 147

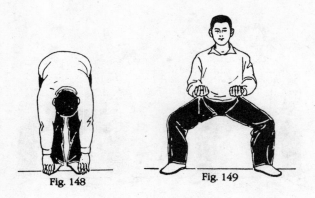

Fig. 148   Fig. 149

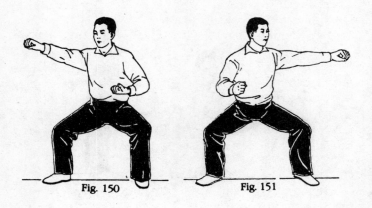

Fig. 150   Fig. 151

102

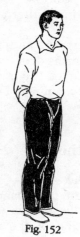

Fig. 152

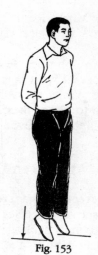

Fig. 153

bent first, then stretched, and left stretched first, then bent. Return to centre, then sway head and torso to right again. Stand erect.

6. Touching Feet with Hands (Figs. 147 and 148)

Stand erect with knees fully extended, legs close together. Bend back with head facing upward, stretch arms behind with hands bent at wrists, palms facing downward pressing hard as if propping on something. Then exhale as you bend forward with arms moving over head and down to touch feet. Stand erect and inhale as you bend back again. Repeat exercise several times.

7. Clenching Fists with Angry Eyes (Figs. 149-151)

Squatting with knees wide apart, clench fists at waist with palms up. Push right fist forward slowly, exhaling, until right arm is straight, with palm facing downward.

103

Gaze forward. Return to original position. Repeat movement with left fist, then continue alternating sides.

8. Rising on Toes Seven Times (Figs. 152 and 153)

Stand erect with legs straight. Let arms drop naturally with palms pressing against front of thighs. Lift heels one to two inches; keep head erect; inhale. Lower heels; exhale. Do seven times.

Eighteen Exercise Methods

A. Prevention and Treatment of Neck Ache

This set of exercises is composed of movements of the head and neck. Exercising the head and upper extremities brings about smooth action of the neck, shoulders, elbows and phalangeal joints, improvement of blood circulation, adjustment of functions of nervous and humoral systems, improvement in the oxidation-reduction processes of muscles and other soft tissues, loosening of spasm and adhesion of these soft tissues, increase in mobility of neck, shoulders, arms and fingers. Digestive and brain functions are also regulated.

1. Shooting Bow on Either Side

Stand erect with feet apart slightly more than shoulder width. Hold hands 30 cm apart in front of face, palms facing forward and thumbs and index fingers pointing towards one another to form a circle. Gaze forward (Fig. 154).

Separate hands and move to sides; make loose fists, facing forward; let elbows drop naturally. Turn head to the left. Gaze past the fist into the distance (Fig.

155). Return to original position.

Do in opposite direction. Do two to four sets of eight.

Points to remember: Don't shrug shoulders when separating hands. Draw shoulder blades together. Keep elbows at even level.

Sensations: In squaring the shoulders and gazing past the fist, you may feel a certain soreness and swelling in the muscles of the neck, shoulders, back and possibly arms. Meanwhile there should be a soothing feeling in the chest.

Effective for aches and stiffness in the neck, shoulders and back, numbness in the arms, depression in the chest, etc.

2. Stretching Arms and Expanding Chest

Stand erect with feet apart slightly more than chest width. Cross hands in front of abdomen with hand on sore side in front, palms facing inward (Fig. 156). Raise arms with eyes gazing at back of the hand on sore side. Return to original position by lowering hands sideways in an arc, the palms first up, then down naturally. Eyes follow hand on sore side (Fig. 157). Do two to four sets of eight.

Points to remember: When raising crossed arms, lift head, thrust out chest and retract abdomen.

Sensations: When raising arms, you may feel soreness in neck, shoulders and waist.

Effective for stiffness and functional disorder of shoulder joints and soreness in neck, back and waist.

3. Stretching One Arm

Stand erect with feet apart slightly more than shoulder width. Stretch left arm sideways and up over head in an arc; gaze at back of left hand. Bend right

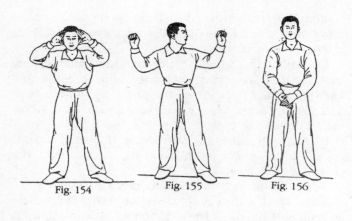

Fig. 154   Fig. 155   Fig. 156

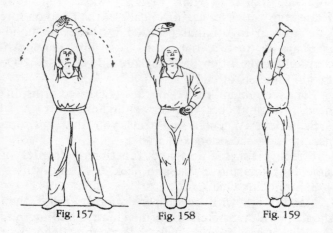

Fig. 157   Fig. 158   Fig. 159

elbow and press the back of right hand on small of back, palm facing out (Figs. 158 and 159). Return to original position. Repeat on opposite side. Do two to four sets of eight.

Points to remember: Stretch arm straight when raising. Keep eyes on raising hand.

Sensations: When stretching the arm upward you may feel soreness in the neck and shoulder on that side and a soothing feeling in the chest.

Effective for stiffness of shoulder joint, pain in the neck, shoulders, back and waist, bloated sensation in stomach.

B. Prevention and Treatment of Lumbago and Backache

This set of exercises is composed of movements of the waist and hips. Exercising the waist, hips and legs will bring about smooth action of the lumbar vertebral and hip joints, improvement in blood circulation, adjustment of the functions of the humoral and nervous systems in the soft tissues of the waist, loosening of spasms and adhesion of these soft tissues, strengthening of muscles in the waist and abdomen, and functinal restoration of abdominal muscles. It is also helpful for checking vertebral malformation, regulating gastrointestinal functions, eliminating distention sensations in the chest and abdomen, strengthening the kidney and nourishing the vital essence.

4. Supporting the Sky with the Hands.

Stand erect with feet apart slightly more than shoulder width. Intertwine fingers in front of abdomen with the palms up (Fig. 160). Raise hands, turning clasped palms upward when passing in front of face,

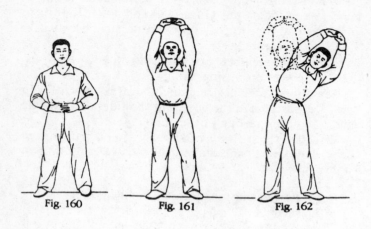

Fig. 160   Fig. 161   Fig. 162

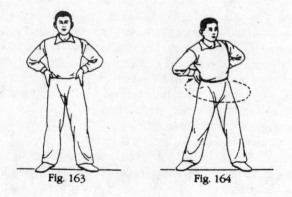

Fig. 163   Fig. 164

then over head; move head back to look at hands (Fig. 161).

Move arms and torso to left. Return to centre and repeat (Fig. 162).

Lower arms sideways and return to starting position. Repeat movements to the right. Do two to four sets of eight.

Points to remember: Keep arms straight and torso erect while turning palms and stretching arms over head.

Sensations: Soreness in the waist and neck, radiating to shoulders, arms and fingers.

Effective for stiffness of the neck and waist, difficulty in motility of shoulders, elbows and vertebral joints, scoliosis of vertebral column.

5. Rotating Torso with Arms Akimbo

Stand erect with feet apart slightly more than shoulder width, arms akimbo with thumbs pointing forward (Fig. 163). Push pelvis forcefully with hands to circle clockwise as far as possible (Fig. 164). Do two sets of eight. Then circle counterclockwise for another two sets of eight.

Points to remember: Circle from small to large until maximum is reached. Stand erect without moving feet. As pelvis moves forward torso inclines backward; push pelvis with both hands to lessen tension of sacrospinal muscles.

Sensations: Marked soreness and distention in lumbar region.

Effective for acute waist sprain and chronic lumbago, hunchback due to occupation or lumbago due to prolonged fixed posture.

6. Touching Feet with Both Hands

Stand erect (Fig. 165). Intertwine fingers in front of abdomen with palms facing upward (Fig. 166). Raise clasped hands, turning palms upward when passing in front of face. Gaze at back of hands (Fig. 167). Straighten back then bend over to touch feet with clasped palms (Fig. 168). Return to starting position. Repeat two to four times.

Points to remember: When bending, move buttocks backward and keep knees straight. Touch feet with as much of the palm as possible.

Sensations: Soreness and distention in the neck and waist when raising the arms, soreness and distention in the legs and waist when bending over and touching feet.

Effective for injuries to soft tissues in legs and waist, vertebral kyphosis, stiffness in waist, numbness and soreness and difficulty in flexing and stretching legs, etc.

C. Prevention and Treatment of Aching Legs and Buttocks

This set of exercises is composed of movements of the legs and buttocks. Exercising the joints of the hips, knees and ankles helps the joints to function smoothly, strengthens the muscles of the waist, abdomen, buttocks and legs, and loosens spasms and adhesions of the soft tissues in the buttocks and legs. Their functions can be increased; malformation of the spinal column and pelvis can be corrected.

7. Rotating the Knees

Stand erect. Bend over with hands touching knees. Gaze at the ground (Fig. 169). Rotate knees clockwise, bending knees on forward movement, straightening

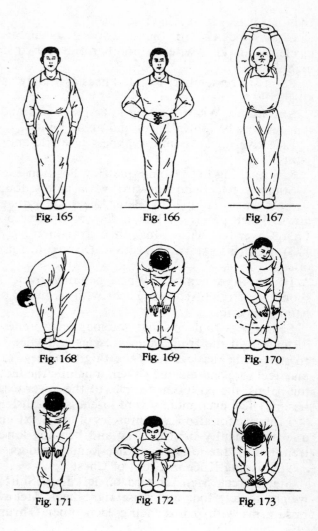

Fig. 165

Fig. 166

Fig. 167

Fig. 168

Fig. 169

Fig. 170

Fig. 171

Fig. 172

Fig. 173

them on backward cycle (Fig. 170).

Circle clockwise for one or two sets of eight, then circle counterclockwise for another one or two sets of eight.

Points to remember: Rotate knees as widely as possible.

Sensations: When rotating knees, soreness and distention may be felt in knees and ankle joints.

Effective for ache and weakness in ankle and knee joints.

8. Stretching Legs from Squatting Position

Stand erect. Bend forward with palms touching straight knees (Fig. 171). Bend knees and squat way down. Place palms on knees, fingers tip to tip (Fig. 172). Cover feet with palms, then straighten legs (Fig. 173). Return to starting position. Do two to four sets of eight.

Points to remember: When bending over, knees should be straight covering feet with as much of the palm as possible.

Sensations: In deep squat you may feel soreness and distention in the front thigh muscles and knee joints. In stretching the legs the back thigh and leg muscles may feel sore and bloated. When touching the feet with the palms, the posterior muscles of the lower extremities may feel even more severe soreness and distention.

Effective for atrophy of muscles of lower extremities due to difficulty in stretching and bending lower extremities or due to hip and knee joint disorders.

9. Hugging Knee in Front of Chest

Stand erect. Step forward on left foot. Shift body weight to left foot and raise right heel. Meanwhile, raise arms with palms facing each other. Thrust out chest and look upward (Fig. 174). Lower arms sideways and raise right knee. Hold close to chest, with left leg straight (Fig. 175). Return to arms upraised position, then to starting position. Repeat on other side. Do two to four sets of eight on either side.

Points to remember: When arms are upraised, body should be kept stable. Press knee as close to chest as possible; supporting leg should be straight.

Sensations: When hugging knee, you may feel soreness and distention in muscles of both supporting leg (posterior part) and raised leg (anterior part).

Effective for soreness of buttocks and legs and difficulty in stretching and bending these parts.

D. Prevention and Treatment of Arthralgia of the Limbs

This set of exercises is composed of movements of the limbs. Exercising the joints of the limbs smooths motions of these joints, eliminates arthralgia, improves the functions of the cardiovascular system and regulative functions of the nervous system. The exercises are helpful for strengthening limb muscles, maintaining their normal shape and loosening adhesion and spasm of soft tissues.

10. Pushing Palm in Leg Rest

Stand erect with feet apart slightly more than shoulder width and with fists clenched at waist. Turn torso to right as far as possible and squat down with right thigh resting on left. Push left palm sideways while looking at right arm (Fig. 176). Return to starting position and do in opposite direction. Do two to four sets of eight.

Points to remember: When squatting, torso should

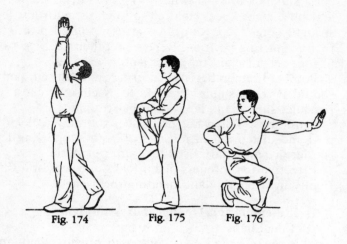

Fig. 174   Fig. 175   Fig. 176

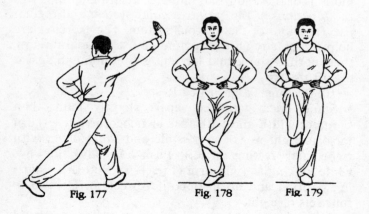

Fig. 177   Fig. 178   Fig. 179

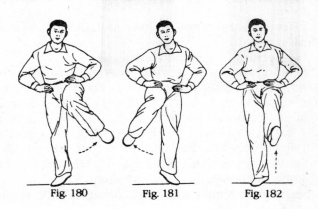

Fig. 180   Fig. 181   Fig. 182

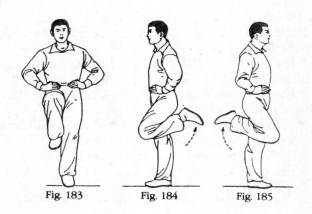

Fig. 183   Fig. 184   Fig. 185

be straight and body weight steady.

Sensations: Soreness and distention in knees, legs and arms.

Effective for soreness in limb joints, neck, back and waist.

11. Turning Torso and Head

Stand erect with feet wide apart and fists clenched at waist. Turn torso to left as far as possible to form a bow step. Gaze over left shoulder. Meanwhile push right palm obliquely upward so that right arm is in line with right leg (Fig. 177). Return to original position and do on opposite side. Do two to four sets of eight.

Points to remember: Keep rear leg straight and heel on ground when performing bow step.

Sensations: Soreness and distention in neck, shoulders and waist.

12. Kicking in All Directions

Stand erect with arms akimbo and thumbs pointing backward. Return to this position after kick.

Raise left knee and kick as if kicking a shuttlecock with inside of left instep (Fig. 178).

Raise right knee and kick as if kicking a shuttlecock with inside of right instep (Fig. 179).

Raise left knee and kick as if kicking a shuttlecock with outside of left instep (Fig. 180).

Raise right knee and kick as if kicking a shuttlecock with outside of right instep (Fig. 181).

Raise left knee and kick forward (Fig. 182).

Raise right knee and kick forward (Fig. 183).

Bend left knee and kick left buttock with heel (Fig. 184). Bend right knee and kick right buttock with heel (Fig. 185).

Point to remember: Keep thigh straight while kicking backward.

Sensations: Soreness and distention in legs.

Effective for pain in hip and knee joints, weakness in legs.

E. Prevention and Treatment of Tenosynovitis

This set of exercise is designed to exercise the shoulder, elbow, wrist and finger joints, improve the blood circulation of the upper-limb soft tissues and the regulation of the nerves and body fluid and ease the adhesion and spasm of the soft tissues of the shoulders, arms and fingers.

13. Pushing Palms in All Directions

Stand erect with feet apart slightly more than shoulder width. Clench fists loosely at waist. Return to this position after each arm movement.

Raise hands above head with palms facing upward, fingertips of left and right hands pointing at each other, thumbs stretched out. Gaze at back of hands (Fig. 186).

Turning torso to left, push arms out on both sides with palms facing outward. Gaze at back of left palm (Fig. 187).

Repeat in opposite direction.

Push arms out on both sides, palms facing outward (Fig. 188).

Do two to four sets of eight.

Points to remember: When turning torso, keep it erect and stand firm without moving feet.

Sensations: Soreness and distention in neck, shoulders, elbows, wrists and fingers.

Effective for tennis elbow, tenosynovitis of the wrist and fingers, soreness in neck, shoulders and waist.

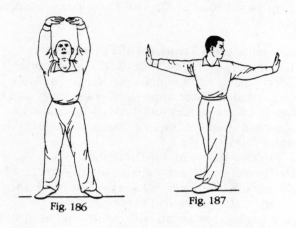

Fig. 186

Fig. 187

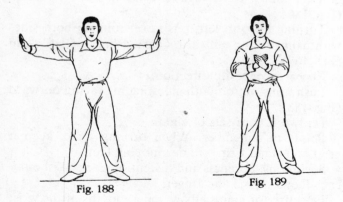

Fig. 188

Fig. 189

118

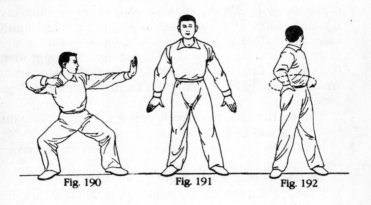

| Fig. 190 | Fig. 191 | Fig. 192 |

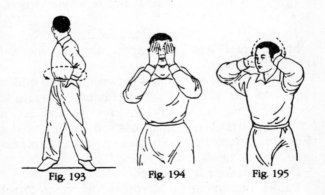

| Fig. 193 | Fig. 194 | Fig. 195 |

14. Drawing a Bow

Stand erect. Step to the left. Cross the hands in front of chest with elbows slightly bent, fingers pointing upward (Fig. 189). Squat slightly and push left hand sideways with palm facing out, fingers pointing up. Gaze at back of left hand. Meanwhile bend right arm in front of chest and jerk elbow back at shoulder level with fist loosely clenched, palm facing downward (Fig. 190).

Loosen fist and press both palms downward as you straighten legs (Fig. 191).

Return to starting position and repeat on opposite side.

Do one or two sets of eight.

Points to remember: During exercise chest should be thrust out. Rotate scapular bone as far back as possible.

Sensations: Soreness and distention in forearms, wrists and back.

Effective for tennis elbow and tenosynovitis of fingers.

15. Relaxing Arms and Turning Torso

Stand erect with feet apart slightly more than shoulder width.

Put the part of right hand between thumb and index finger on left shoulder, palm facing outward. Gaze over left shoulder. Meanwhile press back of left hand on back of waist and turn torso to the left and back (Fig. 192). Return to starting point and repeat on opposite side (Fig. 193).

Do two to four sets of eight.

Points to remember: Drop elbow when touching opposite shoulder with the part of hand between the thumb and index finger and stand still. Movements should be gentle and slow; torso should turn as far as possible.

Sensations: Soreness and distention in neck, shoulders, elbows, wrists and waist.

Effective for rheumatism of shoulder, tennis elbow, waist pain and backache.

F. Prevention and Treatment of Functional Disturbances of Internal Viscera

This set of exercises includes acupoint massage and movements of the trunk and extremities. Blood circulation can be improved, channels dredged, the regulative function of nervous and humoral systems improved. These changes help strengthen cerebral and visceral activities and increase metabolism, thereby producing some therapeutic effect on the heart, liver, spleen, lungs, kidneys, intestines, stomach, etc.

16. Rubbing Face and Kneading Acupoints

Stand erect with feet shoulder width apart. Rub cheeks with middle fingers upward from acupoint *dicang* through *yingxiang*, *bitong* and *jingming* to hairline. (See Chapter IV, "Common Acupoints.") Then, rotating palms, rub downward. Do this eight to sixteen times (Fig. 194).

"Wash" face with palms, moving upward to hairline, then, rotating palms, rub upward to *baihui* point and downward to *fengchi*, around earlobes, back to cheeks, eight to sixteen times (Fig. 195).

Place left palm on upper abdomen. Gaze forward with tongue touching hard palate. Right thumb presses and kneads the *shuimian* point on left hand (at upper third of second metacarpal bone) twenty-four to thirty-six times. Then rub same point on right hand with left thumb the same number of times (Fig. 196).

Points to remember: When rubbing *shuimian* point, close eyes and concentrate the mind. Press palms tight when massaging.

Sensations: Soreness and distention around point when rubbing and warm sensation in cheeks when massaging.

Effective for neurasthenia, insomnia, dizziness, palpitation and gastrointestinal disorders.

17. Turning and Bending Trunk

Stand erect with feet apart and hands clenched at waist level. Raise both hands high above head with palms facing upward, fingers of left and right hands pointing to each other, thumbs separated. Gaze at back of hands.

Lower arms sideways and place hands on waist, arms akimbo, thumbs pointing forward and tips of middle fingers touching each other in back.

Turn trunk leftward as far as possible, eyes gazing in same direction (Fig. 197).

Repeat movements to right (Fig. 198).

Return to centre. Bend forward (Fig. 199).

Stand erect, then lean backward (Fig. 200).

Return to starting position.

Do two to four sets of eight.

Points to remember: When turning trunk, stand firm. When bending forward and back, keep legs straight.

Sensations: Soreness and distension in neck, shoulders and waist.

Effective for weak body, defective kidneys, waist pain and backache.

18. Stretching Arms and Expanding Chest

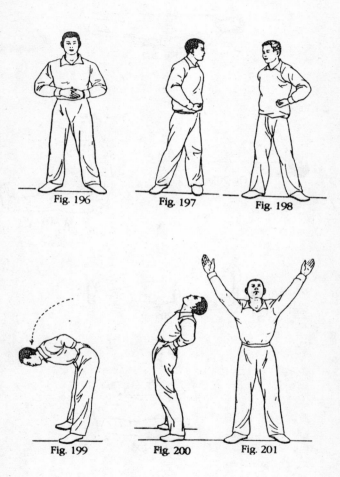

Fig. 196   Fig. 197   Fig. 198

Fig. 199   Fig. 200   Fig. 201

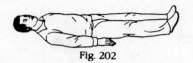

Fig. 202

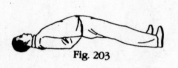

Fig. 203

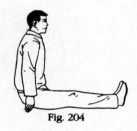

Fig. 204

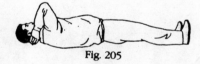

Fig. 205

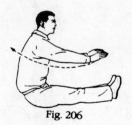

Fig. 206

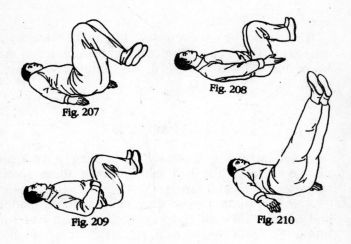

Fig. 207

Fig. 208

Fig. 209

Fig. 210

Stand erect with feet apart. Raise arms, obliquely, crossing when passing in front of trunk, then raise over head in a V as you inhale, lift heels and look upward (Fig. 201). Exhaling and lowering heels, lower arms and cross when passing in front of chest, returning to starting position.

Do two to four sets of eight.

Points to remember: Respiration should be smooth and natural. Gaze at right and left hands alternatly. Raise arms obliquely with strength of forearms.

Sensations: Soreness and distension in neck and shoulders, comfort in chest.

Effective for chronic respiratory and digestive diseases.

Choose any of the exercises, the number depending on your physical condition. All eighteen exercises may be performed until the body is completely rehabilitated.

Bed Exercises

A patient who is seriously ill, extremely weak and unable to leave the bed may practise these special exercises for rehabilitation.

1. Preparations before exercise: Evacuate bladder and bowels. Take off tight clothes. A board bed with pillow half a Chinese foot (about 16 cm.) high is preferable. Lie supine with all muscles relaxed, legs straight and close to each other, arms at small of back. Lie quietly for two minutes (Fig. 202).

2. With support and help of arms at small of back, sit up on bed without moving legs, (Figs. 203 and 204). Lie down as before.

Do movements three or five times.

3. Lie with arms at sides, then, sitting up, raise arms straight beside neck. Bend forward and pull soles of feet with hands around. Do three to five times (Figs 205 and 206).

4. Lie with arms at sides. Raise and bend left arm, then with both hands around back of left knee, draw leg back forcefully, torso and right leg rising naturally; finally, sit up straight with right leg extended straight. Do three to five times on each side.

5. Lie straight with hands flat against bed to support. Raise left bent leg, then raise right leg and bend. Press

both legs against abdomen with force. (Fig. 208). Do three to five times.

6. Lying flat, raise right leg to 45-degree angle then to 90-degree angle. Then raise left leg in same manner. Hold both legs together (Fig. 210). Do one or two times.

Chapter III
Massage Therapy

Brief History

Massage, an integral component of traditional Chinese medicine, is a therapeutic method in which the patients' body or parts of the body are stimulated by massage. Called *pushing and holding* in ancient China, massage was first recorded in the *Yellow Emperor's Internal Classic*. In the chapter "Vital Energy, Blood, Physical and Mental Constitution" it says, "When the body is repeatedly panic-stricken, the channels are impeded. Thus, the body will be numb and should be treated by massage." The famous ancient physician Pian Que applied massage for treating diseases. According to an extant title catalogue the earliest monograph on massage —unfortunately, now lost—was *Ten Chapters on Massage by Huangdi and Qibo*. In the Sui Dynasty (581-618) massage therapy was developed as a special subject. The monograph *On the Etiology and Symptomology of Diseases* (610) mentioned various kinds of massage for treating many diseases. In *Thousand Gold Remedies* Sun Simiao (581-682) of the Tang Dynasty quoted the massage methods proposed by Laozi and Dharmo. *General Collection for Holy Relief* written in 1117 during the Song Dynasty devoted a special chapter to massage therapy. Manipulation and application of massage therapy was further developed in the Yuan Dynasty (1271-1368). The Ming Dynasty established a special department of massage therapy, which was applied extensively in children's diseases. Scores of monographs were published, among them *The Classic of Massage for Children* by Chen of the Siming region and *Secret Principles for Saving Children by Massotherapy* by Gong Yunlin. In the Qing Dynasty *The Golden Mirror of Medicine* (1742) recorded in detail the application of massotherapy in surgery. Since the founding of New China massotherapy has been developed and popularized as an important part of rehabilitation therapy.

Effects

Activation of vital energy and blood, clearing of channels and smoothing of joints. The physical stimulation induced by massage manipulation yields biophysical and biochemical changes in the operated area; the physiological reactions in the local tissues activate and improve lymphatic and blood circulation. Massage causes an increase of the volume of blood flow, which improves the material metabolism of the tissues and the absorption of edema, oozing of blood and old hemorrhage. Since the elasticity of the muscles and ligament is increased, their normal functions can be recovered. Massage also regulates the equilibrium of excitation and inhibition—repeated stimulus produced by mild, rhythmic manipulation induces sedative and inhibitory actions on the nervous system, whereas quick, heavy manipulation excites the nervous system. According to the theory of spinal segmental reflex, massage of the cervical region regulates the blood circulation of the upper limbs and cranium; thus both the intracranial pressure and the blood pressure decrease at the same time. Vibrative and percussive massage of the first and second thoracic vertebrae induces cardiac reflex, manifested by contraction of the cardiac muscles. Vibrative and percussive manipulation of the first and second lumbar vertebrae results in an increase of the volume of blood flow in the minor pelvic cavity. Chiropractic of the spinal column and abdomen speeds up the peristalsis of stomach and intestines. Pressing the supraclavicular acupoints to stimulate the stellate ganglion of sympathetic nerves yields dilatation of the pupils, dilatation of blood vessels and increase of skin temperature of the isolateral side. Massage of the lower abdomen and inner thigh, applied in urine retention, causes contraction of the bladder, resulting in micturition. Abdominal massage causes increase of peristalsis of the intestines and stomach and stimulates secretion of digestive glands. Moreover, after massotherapy, the total leucocyte count increases, with increased phagocytosis and a mild increase of erythrocytes. There are also increases of titre of serum complement, oxygen demands, excretion of nitrogen, urine volume, carbon dioxide, etc.

In brief, massage acts either directly on the impaired organic lesion to eliminate the functional disorder or indirectly by adjusting the functions of the organ to relieve its lesion. It cures organic diseases through the latter mechanism.

Manipulation and Clinical Application

The key element of massage therapy is the various manipulations of the hands or other parts of the body. The effect of the therapy depends on the skill of manipulation and its application. Manipulation must be gentle, even, forceful and persistent, so as to achieve a "penetrating" action. "Gentle" means the manipulation should be light but not superficial, heavy but not sluggish, with no jerking or roughness. "Even" means the manipulation should be rhythmic, neither too quick nor too slow and the pressure should be steady, not sometimes light and sometimes heavy. "Forceful" refers to an optimal strength, varied according to the patient's constitution, disorder, and location of lesion. "Persistent" means the manipulation should last for a definite period without exhausting the patient. All the above points are organically linked to one another. Only after long clinical and manipulation practice can one apply the operation freely, varying it according to the patient's needs.

There are many different massage techniques, and the terminology is not unified. Some techniques have different names for similar movements, and some have similar names but different movements. In treating diseases many methods are generally adopted, supplementing one another. The common basic manipulations are introduced here.

(1) Pushing, including digital and palmar pushing.

Digital pushing: Push a certain part or acupoint of the body with the tip of the thumb. The manipulator should relax shoulder and elbow and raise the wrist. By waving the wrist and flexing and extending the thumb joint pressure is exerted consistently on the acupoint. This is called one-finger pushing (Fig. 211).

Palmar pushing: Press body part with palms and push in one direction (Fig. 212).

Digital pushing is characterized by moderate stimulation of a limited area of contact and is applied at acupoints all over the body, but used mostly for points on the head, face, chest, abdomen and four extremities. It is effective for headache, stomachache, abdominal pain, waist pain and soreness of muscles and joints. Palmar pushing covers a broader contact area and is applied everywhere on the body. The force exerted should be steady and slow. The contact surface should be tightly pressed. Palmar pushing promotes blood circulation in clearing channels.

(2) Holding. Using the thumb in opposition to the index and middle fingers or the other four fingers, the doctor operates on a certain part or acupoint by alternately holding and relaxing the points. (Fig. 213).

Holding is strong stimulation. It is used with other manipulation for points in the neck, shoulders and four extremities. It is usually used as supplementary therapy for stiff neck and sore joints and tendons. Holding should be gentle and continuous, progressing from light to heavy, without any jerking. It eliminates wind and cold, clears channels, soothes muscles, tendons and muscular spasm, etc.

(3) Pressing. Press acupoints or certain parts of the body with the thumb or heel of the palm with increasing force. Press deep with a twisting movement and hold awhile (Fig. 214).

Pressing is a strong stimulator, usually accompanied by rubbing. To do it, clench fist with thumb straight;

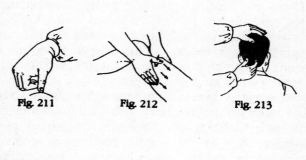

Fig. 211   Fig. 212   Fig. 213

Fig. 214

Fig. 215

Fig. 216

Fig. 217

Fig. 218

use tip or cushion of thumb. When using heel of palm, either one or both palms, overlapping, can be used (Fig. 215). Pressing produces analgesia, relaxes muscles, cures deformities of the spinal cord.

(4) Massaging. Performed by using the palm or the cushion of the index, middle and ring fingers. Press points to be manipulated and massage rhythmically by rotating wrist joint and forearm (Fig. 216).

Massage is gentle stimulation for chest, abdomen and costal parts of the body. It is used for stomachache, abdominal distention, dyspepsia, stagnation of vital energy, etc. When massaging, bend elbow slightly, relax wrist and extend fingers naturally. The cushions of the fingers should rotate with the wrist and forearm. The massaging should be natural, gentle and harmonious, so as to regulate the vital energy and function of stomach-spleen, promote digestion, remove food stagnation and improve peristalsis of the digestive tract.

(5) Rubbing. Press points with palm or ball of thumb (the thenar) and rub to and fro rectilinearly. Rubbing precedes and follows massage therapy (Figs. 217 and 218).

Rubbing, a gentle, warm stimulation, clears channels, activates blood and vital energy, has an antioncotic and analgesic action, regulates digestion, dilates vessels and promotes lymphatic and blood circulation. Rubbing with the palm is usually applied on points of the chest, abdomen and costal region. It is effective for dyspepsia and abdominal ache due to deficiency and cold of the spleen-stomach. Rebbing with the thenar is always applied at shoulders, back, waist, buttocks and lower extremities and is effective for tendon injuries, numbness of the limbs and rheumatic pain and soreness; hypothenar rubbing is always applied to the extremities, chest, abdomen, waist and back and is effective in curing traumatic pain, redness and swelling. All three types of rubbing can be applied freely.

Points to remember: In rubbing, no matter what direction one takes, up and down or left and right, the track should be long, straight without deviation. Rub close to the skin and do not rub hard, so as to avoid bruise.

(6) Slapping. The body is slapped with the palm, fist or a steel racket. Bring the fingers together naturally with the metacarpophalangeal joints slightly flexed. Slap points rhythmically and steadily (Fig. 219). For slapping with the fist, loosely clench fist and use back of fist flat on lesion. For steel racket, use a racket made of steel wire and put a cotton pad covered with cloth (for detail, see Section 4 of this chapter).

Slapping is applied to head, shoulders, back, waist, buttocks and extremities. It is effective for rheumatic soreness, muscle atrophy, cyanosis of the end of limbs, numbness of limbs, and muscular spasm. It harmonizes the vital energy and blood, strengthens bones and tendons, improves blood circulation and eliminates muscle fatigue.

(7) Vibration. Keep forward and back movements even when applying vibration to body. Use fingers or palms, contracting muscles to produce vibration (Fig. 220). Apply vibration to diseased part. Since vibration is tiring, special vibrating instruments have been developed.

Vibration is suitable for all parts of the body. Forcefully contract muscles of forearm and hand and concentrate this strength in the fingertips or palm to

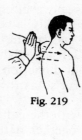

Fig. 219

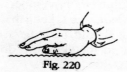

Fig. 220

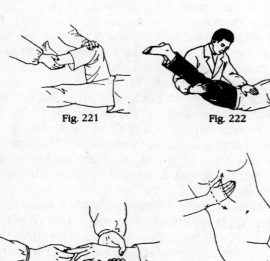

Fig. 221

Fig. 222

Fig. 223

Fig. 224

produce vibration. The vibration should be strong and its frequency high. Usually one hand is used, but sometimes both hands are used at the same time. Vibration acts as an analgesic, activating blood, regulating vital energy and the function of spleen-stomach, promoting digestion and removing food stagnation, regulating digestive functions, etc.

(8) Turning. Hold the distal part of the joint with one hand and the proximal part with the other and gently rotate (Fig. 221).

The method is suitable for treating joints of the four limbs, neck and waist. It is beneficial to motion disorders, stiff joints, and bending and stretching problems. It smoothes articular and tendinous adhesion, loosens the synovial membrane, and strengthens joint movement.

(9) Pulling. Hold the ailing part with both hands or arms, then briskly pull or rotate, moving the hands in opposite directions; the action should produce some noise (Fig. 222).

Movements should be gentle and the force steady. Hands should move cooperatively and synchronously. Clinically, pulling is often used with other methods as an enhancement. It is usually applied to the joints of the neck, shoulders, elbows, wrists, fingers, chest, waist, hips, ankles and vertebrae. It treats body deformity, loosens adhesion and smoothes joints.

(10) Traction. A method often used in dislocation of small joints, tendon injuries, and functional disorders of shoulder or mandibular joints. Traction is used in bone setting for joint dislocations or fracture displacements (Fig. 223).

(11) Rolling. Bend the metacarpo phalangeal joints

slightly. Press the ulnar side of the hand on the part of the body to be treated and shake the heel of the palm rhythmically and continuously by coordinated pronation-supination movements of the forearm and flexion-extension movements of the wrist joint (Fig. 224). The rolling movement exerts force evenly on the part to be treated, clearing channels, stretching and relaxing tendons, activating the vital energy, blood circulation and analgesia.

The following points should be remembered during massage:

1. Usually, massage shouldn't be applied in cases of weak body, severe illness, acute abdominal disease and cancer.

2. Do not apply massage for acute or chronic suppurative inflammation and infectious skin diseases.

3. Don't apply on bleeding areas.

4. Pregnant or menstruating women should not have massage in the waist, lumbosacral plexus or abdomen.

5. It is necessary to guard against fainting if the patient is hungry or has just done vigorous exercise.

Treatment of Common Diseases

1. Stiff neck caused by cold or awkward sleeping position: manipulation by repeated rolling or pushing on the ailing side, together with mild anterior flexing, posterior extension and lateral rotation movements.

Method for treating stiff neck: The patient sits erect. The technician stands opposite, holding the patient's head in his hands and treating him by pulling on the cervical vertebral joints. When pulling the left side, support the right mandible with one hand and hold the left occipital-temporal portion with the other hand. Gently rotate the head ten to twenty times, then turn the head suddenly towards the ailing side and stop. During pulling, a noise may be heard. Movements are the same for the right side only in reverse position. After manipulation, let the patient turn the neck in all directions until he has complete freedom of movement. No further manipulation is needed unless the problem is not cured or alleviated, in which case the manipulation may be repeated one or twice (Fig. 225).

2. Cervical vertebral disease, also known as degenerative disease of the cervical vertebra. It originates in retrograde pathological changes in the intervertebral discs (chronic atrophy of its cervical portion), which worsen as one grows older and strain and trauma increase. When one reaches the age of forty or so, degenerative protrusion of the intervertebral discs appears, with labial hyperplasia of the anterior and posterior borders and hypertrophic changes and semi-dislocation in the small joints. These changes would eventually lead to stricture of the intervertebral foramens, transverse process foramens and spinal canal, which would inevitably stimulate or even oppress the cervical nerve root, vertebral artery, anterior root artery, anterior spinal artery and spinal cord, leading to a series of clinical manifestations, such as pain and numbness of the neck, shoulders, arms, scapular region, upperchest and upper extremities, which are characteristics of chronic, relapsing diseases in old and middle-aged individuals.

Treatment of cervical vertebral disease:

The patient sits erect with his head inclined forward a little to expose the neck fully (a weak patient may assume a prone position with a cushion under the chest). The physician first presses and massages the *du* channel from the *fengfu, yamen* to *dazhui* points with the thumb (mainly on the tender points). Then massage along the bilateral bladder channels from the *tianzhu* and *dashu* tender points to the *jianzhong-shu, jiangwaishu* and *tianzong* points along the Small Intestinal Channel (massage of *tianzong* yields an electric shock sensation). Rolling can be applied to the above points, turning accompanied by traction for the neck. Roll sideways to and fro several times, using light, gentle and slow movements. No sudden force should be used. The extent to which the neck is rotated and the amount of force applied depends on the patient's tolerance. After manipulation a plaster for invigorating blood circulation and eliminating evil wind is applied locally.

Massotherapy, being a kind of rational physiotherapy, is beneficial to the elimination of inflammation and edema, improvement of blood circulation, relief of muscular spasm, prevention of muscular atrophy, increase of muscle tonicity, and amelioration of the function of small joints.

3. Periarthritis of shoulder joint. This is an extensive inflammation of the shoulder region, with marked pain during the night and while resting. Movement of the joint is limited, especially in opening out or in outward rotation. In later stages adhesions occur and the joint becomes a "frozen" shoulder.

Treatment of periarthritis: The operator stands behind the patient, who is sitting erect on a chair. Rolling or pushing is applied to the neck and shoulder regions along with holding or pressing the *jianjing* and *tianzong* points and passive movement of the ailing extremity in and out, in inward and outward rotation, extension, flexion and raising of the arm. In outward rotation, extension, and raising of the arm, move it in circles so as to increase the extent of the joint movement. Use no sudden or violent force. To end the therapy, turn, rub between the hands and shake the shoulder area.

4. Protrusion of lumbar intervertebral discs also called rupture of the fibre ring of the lumbar intervertebral discs. The intervertebral disc is the portion between the vertebral bodies. Clinically, the lumbar fourth and fifth and the lumbar fifth and sacral first discs are most affected.

Treatment: (1) The patient adopts a prone position with no pillow and the head turned to one side. Massage the waist with the heel of the palm, the lumbarsacral region with overlapping palms, the buttocks with a single palm, and the tender points lateral to the lumbar vertebrae with the thumb on either side. Press the lumbar muscles and buttock muscles with separate palms. Strike the buttocks and the length of the leg to the heel with a loose clenched fist. To pull the leg, press the lumbar-sacral region with one hand and support the thigh-knee portion on the opposite side with the other hand so as to extend and abduct the thigh to its greatest extent (Fig. 226). Briskly pull and stretch the leg. Perform the same movements on the opposite side. (2) The patient lies on one side with the lower leg extended and the upper leg flexed. Use the lateral pulling method by pressing down on the lower part of

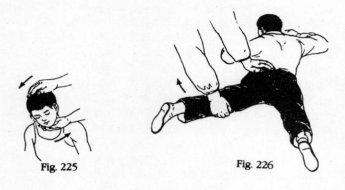

Fig. 225

Fig. 226

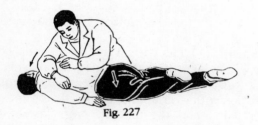

Fig. 227

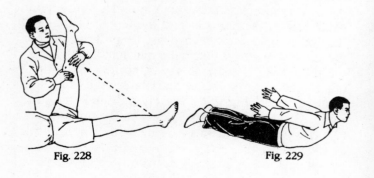

Fig. 228

Fig. 229

the buttocks with one hand or elbow and pressing the anterior of the shoulder-clavicular area with the other hand or elbow. Rotate the waist gradually to its greatest extent (Fig. 227). Then suddenly press down on the waist and relax. Usually a noise can be heard. Do the same movements on the opposite side. (3) The patient lies supine. Test the leg by raising it, extended straight, to high, intermediate and low positions (Fig. 228). Repeat the movements several times. (4) Lastly, have the patient assume a prone position. Massage the waist and buttocks; press and push them several times.

5. Sciatica. Use the same treatment as for protrusion of lumbar intervertebral discs.

6. Waist strain: Denotes chronic injuries of the muscles, ligaments, fasciae, etc. Of the chronic lumbago, lumbar muscle strain constitutes the majority, and the patients are mostly labourers.

Treatment: Similar to protrusion of lumbar intervertebral discs, but whether or not manipulation should be applied depends upon the diagnosis. If the injury is limited to the soft tissue of the waist, rather than the lumbar vertebrae, pulling is unnecessary. For aged people apply gentle massage; avoid pulling. While working, the patient should change positions as much as possible. Bad habits of incorrect posture should be checked. Wearing a wide belt around the waist, and using a board bed are preferable. Exercise the waist muscles by assuming a "fish leap" posture (Fig. 229).

Keep-Fit Massage

(1) Sitting Still (Fig. 230)

Take a freely cross-legged sitting position with the eyes gently closed, the trunk and thighs forming a right angle. Drop shoulders, relax chest, touch tongue tip to hard palate, and clench fists or place hands on the thighs. Breathe naturally for ten minutes, then change to harmonious or reverse breathing for another ten minutes. Sit quietly for twenty to thirty minutes.

Sitting still rests the cerebral cortex cells, helping them recover their function. As a result, the cerebral cortex exerts favourable regulative actions on the organs of the body. Both harmonious and reverse breathing are deep respiration, which improves blood circulation, promotes metabolism, affords a rich oxygen supply, massages the internal organs, improves digestive functions and increases the body's resistance.

(2) Ear Exercise

1. Massage of the auricles: Rub auricles up and down with both palms twenty times.

2. Beating a celestial drum: Cover ears with palms. Put index finger on middle finger, which is on lower margin of occipital bone. Slide index finger down to strike *fengchi* points twenty times. A *"dong, dong"* noise can be heard, like striking a drum (Fig. 231).

3. Drawing the fingers out of the ear: Insert the index finger into the external auditory meatus, then draw it out; do this five times.

Ear exercises strengthen the function of the acoustic nerve, tympanic membrane and auditory tube, promote blood circulation and are good for deafness, tinnitus, dizziness, and body equilibrium. They are unfavourable for acute or chronic inflammation of the ear (Fig. 232).

(3) Mouth Exercises

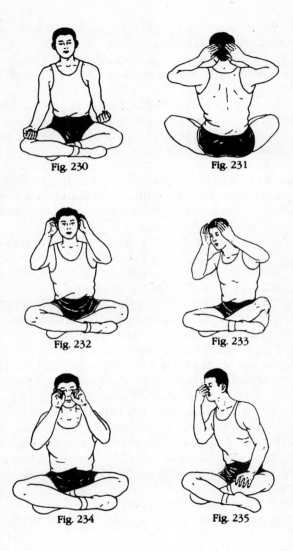

Fig. 230

Fig. 231

Fig. 232

Fig. 233

Fig. 234

Fig. 235

1. Mastication: Concentrate the mind and gently masticate twenty times.

Effects: dilates the vessels of the teeth's roots, promotes blood circulation, hardens the teeth, and prevents tooth diseases.

2. Stirring with the tongue: Rub the tip of the tongue over the inside, outside, left side, right side, top and bottom of the teeth for twenty times. The saliva secreted cleans the mouth. Spit out the first mouthful, then swallow the rest.

Effects: increases the perceptive property of the buccal mucosa and strengthens the secretion function, which stimulates the appetite and promotes digestion.

(4) Eye Exercises

1. Massaging the temples: Massage the temples with the thumbs twenty times (Fig. 233).

2. Massaging eyelids, rotating eyes: Gently close eyes. Rub backs of thumbs together until warm. Gently massage eyelids first, then eyebrows with thumb backs, each twenty times. Rotate eyes, first clockwise, then counterclockwise, each ten times (Fig. 234).

3. Pinching bridge of nose: Put index finger on the *xuanguan* point between the eyebrows. Pinch bridge of nose with middle finger and thumb at greater canthus on both sides twenty times (Fig. 235).

The gentle, warm massage adjusts the nerves, promotes blood circulation, stimulates the lacrimal secretion that protects and lubricates the eyeballs. Rotating the eyeballs exercises the muscles and increases flexibility, preventing eye-muscle fatigue and strengthening vision.

(5) Nose: Pressing the *Yingxiang* Points

First rub backs of lower part of thumbs together

until warm, then press along sides of nose twenty times. Then press *yingxiang* points (in nasal-labial groove) with tips of index fingers in circular way ten times.

Effects: promotes blood circulation of nasal mucosa, increases nasal secretion for wetting nasal cavity, prevents dust from passing through cavity and acts as a filter. Good for preventing and treating rhinitis.

(6) Dry "Washing" of Face

Rub palms together, until warm, then rub face from forehead downward along cheeks and upward from mouth to forehead. Up and down do twenty times (Fig. 236).

Effects: improves blood circulation in face, giving ruddy appearance, increases elasticity of facial muscles and skin and activity of nerves, increases sight, strengthens teeth, decreases wrinkles and produces other cosmetic effects.

(7) Combing the Scalp

Hook fingers and comb scalp with nails first on apex, secondly on "horn part" of the parietal bone, thirdly on temporal and lateral parts each for ten times. Then massage scalp with palms twenty times (Fig. 237).

Effects: promotes blood circulation of scalp. Prevents and treats headache and dizziness and clears the head.

(8) Neck Exercises

1. Stroking head and neck: Interlace fingers to embrace neck from behind with head inclining backward and eyes looking upward. Inhale through nose at same time. Then drop head forward and downward, exhaling through nose. Stroke neck to and fro ten times (Fig.238).

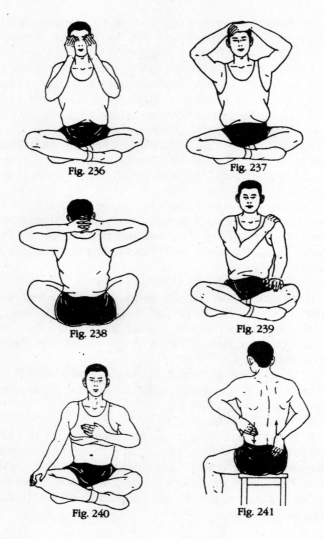

Fig. 236

Fig. 237

Fig. 238

Fig. 239

Fig. 240

Fig. 241

148

2. Looking sidewards: Turn head looking first to the left, then to the right twenty times.

Effects: Local massage and muscular movement of neck and shoulders help prevent and treat stiff and sore neck.

(9) Kneading Shoulders

Knead each shoulder with opposite palm twenty times (Fig. 239).

Effects: improves local blood circulation, preventing inflammation of the shoulder region.

(10) Stroking Chest

Rub palms until warm, then place left palm on right chest and rub up and down fifty times (Fig. 240). Do on opposite side. Then pound right chest with left fist or palm three times moving downward; pound left chest with right fist or palm. Do a total of one hundred times.

Effects: improves blood circulation, increases vital capacity, develops tendons of chest, increases movements of internal viscera.

(11) Rubbing Waist

Rub palms until warm, then rub waist up and down with warm palms twenty times. (Fig. 241).

Effects: good for preventing and treating waist pain. Local massage improves blood circulation and eliminates stagnant blood. Affects lumbar-sacral nerves and strengthens, through reflex action, innervating organs, thus preventing and curing waist pain, kidney deficiency, lumbar muscles strain and dysmenorrhoea.

(12) Rubbing the *Dan Tian* point (also called *Qihai*, below the navel)

Rub palms until warm. Place right palm on abdominal wall near navel. Press right hand with left palm, then, press abdomen with overlapping hands, moving along tract of large intestine around navel, from lower right to upper right, to upper left, to lower left part of abdomen. Do a hundred cycles (Fig. 242).

Prevents and cures dyspepsia and constipation.

3. Rubbing the scrotum: Rub palms until warm, then rub the *dan tian* point with one palm and carry the scrotum up and down with the other. Do eighty-one times with each hand. This exercise is recorded in an ancient work saying: "Rub and carry changing hands, nine times nine. This will retain the *yang* principle." This exercise cures emission, premature ejaculation and impotence.

(13) Twisting the *Weizhong* Point

Twist the left *weizhong* point with the right thumb and the right point with the left. Do twenty times. Prevents and cures waist pain and backache.

(14) Rubbing the *Yongquan* Point

Rub centre of right sole with left hand and left sole with right hand. It is best to rub until centre of soles warm or slightly perspiring. Good for preventing and curing hypertension. However, it should be emphasized that for hypertension, it is preferable to rub forward instead of to and fro, as indicated for other ailments (Fig. 243).

(15) Rowing a Boat

Sit erect on a board bed with both legs extended and toes pointing upward. Palms facing outward, push over legs towards feet, inclining trunk forward and exhaling until above feet. Draw hands back, palms facing inward, inhaling and leaning back. Do twenty times. Increases vital capacity and regulates blood circulation (Fig. 244).

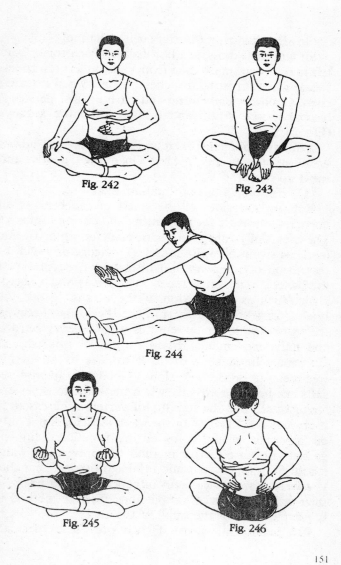

Fig. 242

Fig. 243

Fig. 244

Fig. 245

Fig. 246

(16) Harmonizing the *Dai* (belt) Channel

Sit with legs crossed. Clasp hands. Turn torso from left to right ten times, then from right to left ten times. Inhale when thrusting out chest; exhale when relaxing chest. Good for preventing and curing waist pain and lumbar muscle strain and for strengthening kidneys (Fig. 245).

After finishing the exercise, sit quietly and adjust breathing for twenty cycles. Open eyes gently and stand up slowly.

(17) Rubbing Sides of Small of Back

Rubbing the sides of the small of the back is an important measure for preventing and curing lumbago. The causes of lumbago are varied, including myogenic (such as strain of waist muscles), osteogenic (such as protrusion of intervertebral discs and hyperplasia of the bones), neurogenic (such as sciatica) and viscerogenic (such as retroflexion of the uterus). Since the lumbar vertebrae and sacrum are the bridge between the trunk and lower extremities with a heavy burden and active movements, they are apt to be injured.

Chronic lumbago is difficult to cure by allopathic treatment or medicines alone. Good therapeutic results can be achieved only when the waist muscles are strengthened and the stability of vertebra increased. It is obvious that exercise of the waist muscles is not only an important measure for curing functional lumbago but also an effective method for preventing waist strain. Sufferers of chronic lumbago (except that due to tuberculosis, cancer and infection) should exercise their waist muscles. A simple and effective method is to rub the sides of the small of the back.

Rub palms until warm. Tightly press sides of small

of back with palms and rub downward to coccyx forcefully. Return upward as high as possible. Do fifty to a hundred times (Fig. 246).

Clench fists loosely and beat small of back with edge of fists. Or massage points with back of fists. One may also pinch waist muscles along edge of sacrum. Pinch up and down ten times. Use thumb and middle finger to lift muscles. Push muscles down with thumb above and index and middle fingers underneath so as to make them "roll." Pinch once or twice daily for good results.

Coordinating "bending trunk to move feet by hands" movements, either bending or rotating the waist, is more effective.

In TCM it is recognized that the small of the back is the convergent point of the vital gates of the *du* channel, the *shenshu* of the urinary bladder channel and the *dai* (belt) channel and is the essential root of one's being. Rubbing the small of the back nourishes genuine vital energy, harmonizes blood and vital energy, clears vessels and channels, reinforces tendons and bones, stops pain and eliminates evil wind. It possesses rehabilitative action and is effective in preventing and curing functional lumbago, especially chronic strain of waist muscles and acute waist sprain. It is also effective in hyperplasia of bone tissue, protrusion of intervertebral discs, sciatica, etc.

Chiropractic

Chiropractic, a simple and effective folk rehabilitative therapy, is an operation performed on the back of the patient for curing diseases.

For children it is mainly effective for dyspepsia and digestive disorders (loss of appetite, vomiting, abdominal distension, diarrhoea and constipation), infantile malnutrition, nocturia, insomnia, etc. For adults it is effective for insomnia, drowsiness, acute and chronic gastritis, acute and chronic enteritis, chronic hepatitis, neurasthenia, hypertension, lumbago, etc.

Method: the patient assumes a prone position. The operator uses both hands in loose fists, pinching the skin with the thumb below the skin and the fingers above it, pushing the skin with the thumb towards the head, while drawing it back with the fingers making the skin pinched as if rolling along the spinal column from the coccyx upward to the *dazhui* point of the cervical vertebrae. Do seven times. In severe cases the movements may be supplemented by chiropractic of the urinary bladder channels along both sides of the spinal column another seven times for favourable results. After these, select different points for different diseases (*pishu* point for dyspepsia, *xinshu* point for insomnia, *shenshu* point for lumbago and hypertension), pinch and lift the skin forcefully for three times. To end, massage the pinched point one or two minutes (Figs. 247 and 248).

Points to remember: 1. For pinching movements the two hands should have even strength. The skin pinched should have proper thickness and the pinching action proper tightness. Generally, 0.5 to 1 cm of skin is pinched. 2. As a rule, about ten seconds for one session of chiropractic is appropriate. 3. Not appropriate for skin infection. 4. For loss of appetite, pinch before eating a meal; for dyspepsia, distension of abdomen and stuffy chest after a meal. 5. During summer, when

Chiropractic Chart (1)

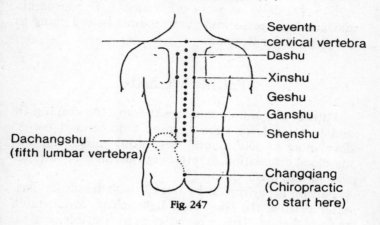

Seventh cervical vertebra
Dashu
Xinshu
Geshu
Ganshu
Shenshu

Dachangshu (fifth lumbar vertebra)

Changqiang (Chiropractic to start here)

Fig. 247

Chiropractic Chart (2)

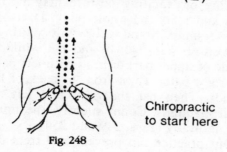

Chiropractic to start here

Fig. 248

155

the back is sweaty, it must be dried with a towel first, then sprinkled with talcum powder to avoid slippery skin. 6. Do daily or every other day. 7. For insomnia and nocturia, performing chiropractic before going to bed is good for sleeping.

Patting Methods

Patting is a simple massage therapy for keeping fit and is helpful for strengthening tendons and bones, developing muscle tissues, lubricating joints, improving blood circulation, reinforcing functions of internal viscera and metabolism.

Patting is performed by oneself with hands or fists. After patting, the body feels light, clear, comfortable and quickened. This method is more flexible, active, practical and effective than passive massage. Patting with a racket made of steel wire or a sand bag is also effective.

1. Patting the Head

A walking or standing posture may be assumed. Stand still and relax the whole body. Drop shoulders and elbows; smile. Stand still while patting. For a walking posture, walk slowly and pat while walking. Pat left side of upper part of head with left palm, right side with right palm, from front to back of head, for fifty rounds. Then pat the right and left sides for another fifty rounds. Count silently, the mind calm, breathing naturally (Figs. 249 and 250).

Persistent practice can prevent and treat dizziness, headache, insufficient blood supply, etc.

2. Patting Upper Extremities

Starting position same as before. Pat four sides of left arm from above downward, patting each side twenty-five rounds (divided into five times, each five rounds). Pat right arm for a total of one to two hundred rounds (Figs. 251 and 252).

Prevents or relieves poor muscle growth of upper extremity, cyanosis of the end of limbs, numbness of upper extremity, hemiplegia, etc.

3. Patting Both Shoulders

Starting position same as before. First, pat left shoulder with right palm, then pat right shoulder with left palm. Pat alternately for fifty to one hundred rounds (Figs. 253 and 254).

Prevents and cures inflammation of perishoulder tissues, frozen shoulder, underdevelopment of muscles, atelectasis, etc.

4. Patting Back

Starting posture same as before. Pat left side of back with right fist, right side of back with left fist, each one to two hundred times (Figs. 255 and 256).

Prevents and cures backache, chronic bronchitis, pulmonary emphysema, atelectasis, underdevelopment of muscles, coronary heart disease, arteriosclerosis, etc.

5. Patting Chest

Alternately pat chest with opposite fist or palm. Pat downward, then upward. Do one to two hundred rounds on each side (Figs. 257 and 258).

Prevents and cures coronary arteriosclerotic heart disease, hypertensive heart disease, rheumatic heart disease, pulmonary emphysema, cor pulmonale, underdevelopment of muscles, etc.

6. Patting Waist and Abdomen

Pat with palms or fists. Move upper extremities by

157

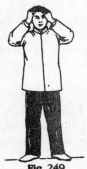

Fig. 249

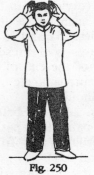

Fig. 250

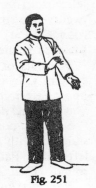

Fig. 251

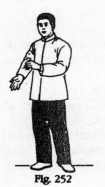

Fig. 252

Fig. 253

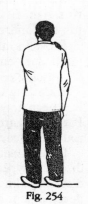

Fig. 254

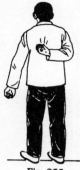

Fig. 255

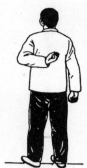

Fig. 256

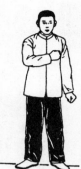

Fig. 257

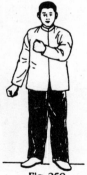

Fig. 258

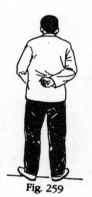

Fig. 259

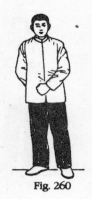

Fig. 260

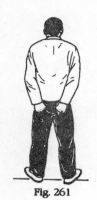

Fig. 261

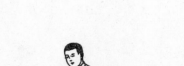

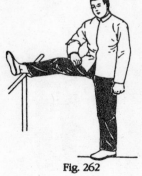

Fig. 262

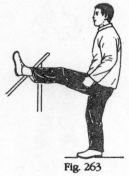

Fig. 263

rotating torso on waist axis and pat left abdomen with right hand, right side of small of back with left hand; then switch side. Pat upper, middle and lower side of small of back. Do one to two hundred rounds on each side (Figs. 259 and 260).

Prevents and cures soreness of waist, lumbago, hyperplasia of bones, dyspepsia, abdominal distention, constipation, etc.

7. Patting Buttocks

Pat left buttock with left palm or fist and right buttock with right hand or fist. Do fifty to a hundred times (Fig. 261).

Prevents and cures sciatica, atrophy of hip muscles, hypoplasia, numbness, etc.

8. Patting Legs

Stand erect. Raise left leg so thigh and lower leg form right angle. Rest heel of left foot on support (such as a tree branch or fence). Slap leg from thigh towards foot on all four sides. Do five to ten times on each side, each time containing one to two hundred rounds, five beats for each round. Do the same on opposite side.

Prevents and cures maldevelopment of leg muscles, hemiplegia, paraplegia, cyanosis of leg, numbness and myasthenia of leg, difficulty in lifting feet when walking (Figs. 262 and 263).

Remarks: When patting, go from light to heavy and do it consistently.

Chapter IV

Acupuncture-Moxibustion and Other Therapeutic Methods

Acupuncture-Moxibustion Therapy

Acu-moxibustion, an art in TCM with a history of thousands of years, is a combination of acupuncture and moxibustion, two independent healing arts. Acupuncture refers to the use of metal needles (in ancient times needles were made of stone) on certain points of the body for regulation of vital energy, blood, nutrients and defensive energy. Moxibustion refers to the application of burnt or heating materials on body points for warming up the blood and energy to facilitate the flow, supporting the *yang* principle and eliminating cold. Clinically, the two therapies are always applied together.

(1) Origin and Evolution
In the earliest extant medical work, *The Yellow Emperor's Canon of Internal Medicine,* composed of two parts: the *Plain Question* and *Miraculous Pivot,* each in nine volumes, believed to have been written during the Warring States Period in the fifth century B.C., acupuncture and moxibustion are mentioned. All

the famous physicians of successive ages recorded and
developed the art of acu-moxibustion therapy, including Zhang Zhongjing's *On Febrile Diseases* and *Synopsis of the Golden Cabinet* of the Han Dynasty (third
century), Fu Weng's *Classic of Acupuncture and Pul-
sology* of the Late Han Dynasty (third century),
Huangfu Mi's (215-282) *A Classic of Acupuncture and
Moxibustion* (282) of the Jin and Southern and North-
ern dynasties, Sun Simiao's (581-682) *Thousand Gold
Remedies for Emergencies* and *A Supplement to "Thou-
sand Gold Remedies"* (652) of the Tang Dynasty, Wang
Tao's *Medical Secrets of an Official* (752) of the Tang
Dynasty, Wang Weiyi's *Illustrated Manual on the
Points for Acupuncture and Moxibustion as Found on
the Bronze Figure* (1026) of the Song Dynasty, Wang
Zhizhong's *Acupuncture and Moxibustion Classic for
Keeping Fit* (752) of the Song Dynasty, Dou Hanqing's
A Guide to Acupuncture and Moxibustion (1115) of the
Liao-Jin-Yuan dynasties, Hu Tai Bi Lie's *Jin Lan Sun's
Classic* (1308), Hua Boren's *Expounding of Fourteen
Channels* (1341), Wang Guorui's *Jade Dragon's Clas-
sic of Acupuncture and Moxibustion by Bian Que*
(1368) of the Jin-Yuan dynasties, Xu Feng's *The Com-
plete Works of Acupuncture and Moxibustion* (1439),
Weng Ji's *Questions and Answers on Acupuncture and
Moxibustion* (1530), Gao Wu's *The Collection of the
Best in Acupuncture and Moxibustion* (1529), Yang
Weizhou's *Compendium of Acupuncture and Moxibustion* (1601), Li Pinhu's *Research on Eight Extraordi-
nary Channels* (1640) of the Ming Dynasty, Li Shou-
xian's *Easy Mastery of Acupuncture and Moxibustion*
(1798) and Li Xuechuan's *Easy Approach to Acupuncture and Moxibustion* (1817) of the Qing Dynasty. All

these works played an important role in the development of acu-moxibustion and its application.

Acupuncture-moxibustion has not only made great contributions to health care in China but it also spread to Japan and Korea as early as the fifth century and to France, Italy and Germany in about the seventeenth century. Currently it has become the focus of attention, especially since extensive application of this healing art has led to a new field, acupuncture analgesia, which is in high repute both at home and abroad.

(2) Relations Between Body Channels and Acu-moxibustion

Channels, or meridians, the passages for the flow of blood and vital energy, originate in the internal viscerae both hollow and solid, and spread all over the tissues and organs of the body. Through channels the organs are closely connected, either directly or indirectly and interrelated. Hence, disorders of one organ might spread to another organ and, similarly, disease in the interior might reflect on the surface of the body, while stimulation of the body's surface might affect internal organs. This rule is true both physiologically and pathologically. By applying this theory or hypothesis, TCM doctors observe and cure diseases with acu-moxibustion.

(3) Methods

(a) Puncturing with filiform needle

1. Holding the needle

Though there are different ways of holding the needles, the common method is to hold the handle of the needle with right thumb and index finger, support-

Fig. 264

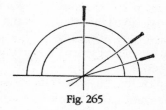

Fig. 265

ing the body of the needle with middle finger, with one or two *fen* (a *fen* equals 1/3 centimetre) left uncovered, just like holding a Chinese writing brush. The puncturing is quick and accurate with little or no pain (Fig.264).

2. Direction of puncturing

Varies according to the thickness of the muscle (Fig. 265).

a. Perpendicular puncturing: puncture perpendicularly (a ninety-degree angle between the needle and skin). Mostly applied to points on the limbs and to thick muscles.

b. Oblique puncturing: puncture obliquely at an angle fifty to sixty degrees between needle and skin.

c. Transverse puncturing, also called puncturing along the skin: puncture transversely along the skin's surface at an angle ten to twenty degrees between needle and skin. Mostly applied on points where muscle is quite thin or when the needle penetrates several points. It is not appropriate for manipulation with great amplitude, such as the *baihui* and *shangxing* points.

3. Method of inserting needle

a. Slow twisting insertion: Keeping tip of needle pointing to the point (avoiding hair pores) perpendicularly, twist needle. At same time insert into skin by pressing twisting needle. Twist angle shouldn't exceed ninety degrees, and inserting should be as quick as possible.

b. Rapid insertion: Press skin to be punctured with left hand and, holding needle in right hand, point accurately at acupoint and quickly insert into skin. Commonly applied for short filiform and three-edged needles.

c. Twist insertion: Wrap body of needle with cotton, leaving one to two *fen* of tip uncovered. Accurately and repidly pierce skin, the left hand protecting the needle, the right hand holding the handle. Twist needle at the same time as piercing. Applied on points where muscles are thick and abundant and long needles are used.

In brief, the key to inserting is twisting and pressing.

4. Assisting manipulation

Usually both hands are used in puncturing. The operator holds the needle in his right hand, the "puncturing hand," and is assisted by left hand, the "pressing hand." The pressing hand stretches the skin for puncturing, keeps long needles from bending, decreases pain, and helps induce needle sensation quickly.

There are two methods of manipulating pressing hand:

(1) Nail pressing: press points to be punctured with left thumb nail or left index finger nail. Hold needle in right hand near left nail (without touching). Pierce quickly. Usually applied for short needles (Fig. 266).

(2) Coordinated pressing: Hold needle just above tip with left thumb and index finger (may wrap with

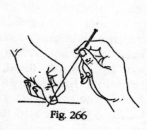

Fig. 266

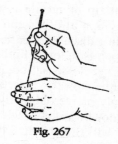

Fig. 267

cotton). Hold body of needle in right hand; pierce skin, twist and press at same time. Applied for long-needle puncturing, such as puncturing of *huantiao* point (Fig. 267).

(3) Stretch pressing: Stretch skin near acupoint and make local skin tense for puncturing. Applied to loose parts of skin and abdominal points.

(4) Holding-tense pressing: Hold skin to be punctured tense by stretching between left thumb and index finger. Pierce skin along surface. Applied in piercing points on thin muscle such as *yintang* point.

5. Depth for puncturing

Varies according to place to be punctured and patient's physique. Piercing may be deeper for fat patient, shallower for thin patient. Points on back and chest are usually pierced shallowly—first pierce two to three *fen*, then transversely along the skin's surface. A deep puncture may result in injury. For points on the limbs a deeper puncture is preferable. Penetrating puncturing should be applied where possible.

6. Controling the direction of needling sensation. The sensation should spread from the puncturing point towards the diseased site. To control the direction,

point tip of needle towards ailing site; at same time press skin at other end of needle in opposite direction against diseased location. For instance, when needling acupoints in lower limbs for treating abdominal disease and needle sensation is induced by perpendicular or oblique upward insertion, turn tip towards torso, or simply pierce obliquely in abdominal direction, pressing downward skin with left hand. The needling sensation will thus be directed upward to the diseased location. Strengthen the stimulation at this time and the sensation will definitely be felt. A sensitive patient is apt to feel the needling conduction, while an insensitive one isn't. For the latter, a local sensation of soreness, numbness, distension or heaviness is enough.

7. Retention of needle after insertion

After needling sensation is felt, leave needle in place without holding for fifteen to twenty minutes, depending on the condition to be treated. For instance, for acute stomachache, convulsions, or appendicitis the duration may be longer, while for critical cases, such as infantile paralysis, no retention is necessary.

8. Withdrawal of needle

After manipulation or retention the needle may be withdrawn in three ways:

(1) Light twisting and lifting: Twist and retain alternately until final withdrawal.

(2) Gradual withdrawal: When patient is at ease with no feeling of heaviness or tenseness, withdraw needle steadily.

(3) Rapid withdrawal with vibrating: Vibrate the needle perpendicularly and withdraw needle rapidly. Applied in emergency cases and for paralytic patients.

9. Frequency of needling.

(1) Acute cases: Needle daily, ten sessions for one course, with a lapse of three to seven days before beginning another course.

(2) Chronic cases: Needle every other day, ten sessions for one course, with a rest of seven days.

(b) Moxibustion

Two common methods of moxibustion are:

1. Ignited moxa cone: A moxa cone is made of moxa wool as large as half a date pit, or a grain of wheat. Glue a ginger or garlic slice to the acupoint and place the moxa cone on tip. Ignite the cone at its tip. The fire will gradually burn downward until the cone is completely consumed. Supply another cone. The warmth penetrates the slice to reach the acupoint. Cones serve as measuring units for moxa treatment. One session of moxibustion may use several or scores of cones.

2. Ignited moxa cylinder: With paper, roll moxa wool into a cylinder. Burn cylinder at one end, and hold the cylinder with the burning end close above the points. Remove to another point after a scorching sensation is felt. Control temperature by varying distance between cylinder and skin. Avoid burning skin. Cylinder moxibustion requires a longer time to produce a sensation—usually fifteen minutes, although it may take much longer.

Effective for rheumatic arthritis, rheumatoid arthritis, gout, pleuritis, facial paralysis, hemiplegia, etc.

CHARTS OF MAJOR ACU-POINTS

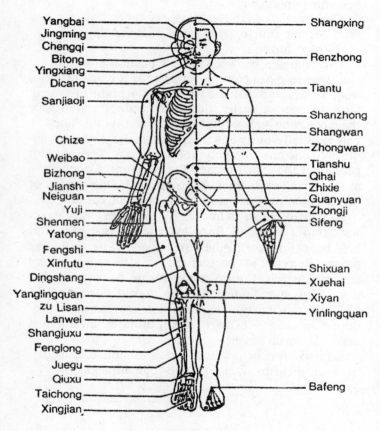

Yangbai
Jingming
Chengqi
Bitong
Yingxiang
Dicang
Sanjiaoji

Chize
Weibao
Bizhong
Jianshi
Neiguan
Yuji
Shenmen
Yatong
Fengshi
Xinfutu
Dingshang
Yanglingquan
zu Lisan
Lanwei
Shangjuxu
Fenglong
Juegu
Qiuxu
Taichong
Xingjian

Shangxing
Renzhong
Tiantu
Shanzhong
Shangwan
Zhongwan
Tianshu
Qihai
Zhixie
Guanyuan
Zhongji
Sifeng
Shixuan
Xuehai
Xiyan
Yinlingquan
Bafeng

Front View

Fig. 268

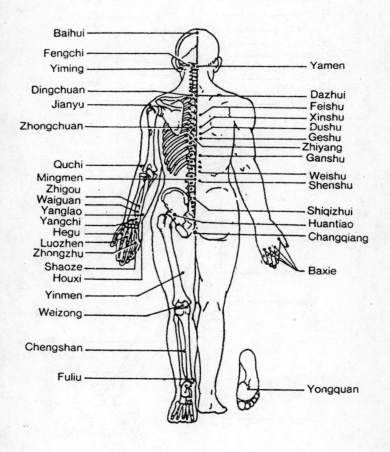

Baihui
Fengchi
Yiming
Dingchuan
Jianyu
Zhongchuan
Quchi
Mingmen
Zhigou
Waiguan
Yanglao
Yangchi
Hegu
Luozhen
Zhongzhu
Shaoze
Houxi
Yinmen
Weizong
Chengshan
Fuliu

Yamen
Dazhui
Feishu
Xinshu
Dushu
Geshu
Zhiyang
Ganshu
Weishu
Shenshu
Shiqizhui
Huantiao
Changqiang
Baxie
Yongquan

Back View
Fig. 269

171

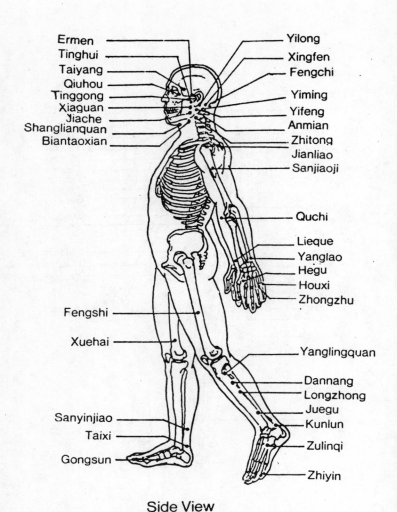

Ermen
Tinghui
Taiyang
Qiuhou
Tinggong
Xiaguan
Jiache
Shanglianquan
Biantaoxian

Yilong
Xingfen
Fengchi
Yiming
Yifeng
Anmian
Zhitong
Jianliao
Sanjiaoji

Quchi

Lieque
Yanglao
Hegu
Houxi
Zhongzhu

Fengshi

Xuehai

Yanglingquan

Dannang
Longzhong
Juegu
Kunlun
Zulinqi

Sanyinjiao
Taixi
Gongsun

Zhiyin

Side View
Fig. 270

172

Common Acupoints (Figs. 268-270)

Part of body	Name	Location	Indications	Method
	Baihui	7 *cun* above posterior hairline, midway on line connecting two apexes of ears	Critical cases, headache, dizziness, prolapse of the anus, hypertension	Sit erect; transverse puncturing forward or backward for 0.5 to 1.5 *cun**
	Shangxing	1 *cun* above anterior hairline, on the mid-sagittal line of head	Headache, pain in eyes, epistaxis, nasal obstruction, rhinitis	Oblique puncturing for 2 to 3 *fen***
	Yangbai	1 *cun* above midpoint of eyebrows	Facial paralysis, nystagmus, itching and pain in eye, trigeminal neuralgia	Oblique puncturing for 3 to 5 *fen*
	Yintang	Midpoint between eyebrows	Headache, pain in eye, pain in nose, dizziness, insomnia, convulsion in children	Pinch skin around point; oblique puncturing from above downward for 0.5 to 1 *cun*

*cun 1/3 decimetre
**fen 1/3 centimetre

173

Jingming	1 *fen* above inner canthus	Conjunctivitis, myopia, glaucoma and other eye diseases	Patient sits erect, with eyes gazing forward. Fix eye ball operated on with left thumb and push sideways. Puncture directly along margin of orbit for 0.5 to 1 *cun* without twisting. A minute filiform needle is preferable to avoid internal bleeding. Push very gently with only light trembling. Press point after withdrawal of needle
Qiuhou	On lower ridge of eye orbit at juncture of outer inner three quarters	Glaucoma, optic neuritis, optic atrophy, vitreous opacity	Puncture obliquely towards optic foramen for 1 to 1.5 *cun*. Patient looks upward when being operated upon.
Chengqi	7 *fen* directly below pupil	Myopia, keratitis, optic atrophy	Push tip of needle towards inner angle
Bitong (Shang-ying-xiang)	1 *cun* above *yingxiang* point, at hollow below nasal bone	Rhinitis, obstruction of nasal ventilation, boil on face, upper toothache, trigeminal neuralgia.	Puncture obliquely upward and medially for 5 to 6 *fen*. A reverse "V" shape is formed when both points are punctured.
Yingxiang	5 *fen* lateral to nostrils, in nasallabial groove	Nasal disorders, facial paralysis.	Also for biliary ascariasis when punctured through to *sibai* point Puncture obliquely towards medial side for 1 *fen* to 1 *cun*

Renzhong	At juncture of upper third lower two thirds philtrum	Syncope, heat stroke, hysteria, swelling and pain in face, hypotension	Puncture obliquely upward and medially. For pain in spinal column, 1/2 to 1 cun; for angina, puncture for several sessions; if ineffective, repeat puncture or let blood with a 3-edged needle.
Dicang	4 fen lateral to corner of mouth	Swelling of face, facial paralysis, profuse salivation	Transverse puncture for 3 fen to 2 cun; may be pushed through to jiache or shangyingxiang points.

Head and Neck

Taiyang	The depression 1 cun behind midpoint between end of eyebrow and lateral canthus	Headache, migraine, eye diseases	Transversely 2 to 3 fen, or obliquely backwards 8 fen to 3 cun
Xiaguan	On lower border of zygomatic arch—a depression when mouth closed	Toothache, mandibular arthritis, lockjaw, facial paralysis	Perpendicularly 0.5 to 1 cun
Yifeng	The depression posterior to ear lobe	Tinnitus, deaf-mutism, swelling of face, trismus, toothache	Lateral-posterior towards medial-anterior 1.5 to 2 cun. Open mouth wide when puncturing.
Yilong	5 fen above yifeng, depression between mastoid process and external ear (auricle)	Deafness	Puncture towards external auditory meatus 5-8 fen
Anmian	Midpoint between yifeng and yiming	Insomnia, schizophrenia.	Perpendicularly 1.5 to 2 cun

Yiming	On lower margin of mastoid process, 1 cun behind yifeng	Optic neuritis, parotitis, cataract, insomnia	Perpendicularly 0.5 to 1.5 cun.
Xingfen	On upper margin of mastoid process	Somnolence	Perpendicularly 5 fen, then turn medially at 45 degree angle and push 1.5 to 2 cun forward
Ermen	In depression anterior to supratragic notch	Deafness, tinnitus, toothache	Perpendicularly 1 to 1.5 cun with the patient's mouth open, or towards larynx 2 cun.
Tinggong	Anterior to tragus; depression formed when mouth open	Deafness, tinnitus, toothache, trigeminal neuralgia, facial paralysis.	Perpendicularly 2 cun; or towards larynx 2 cun
Fengchi	Depression just lateral to neck muscle below occipital bone	Headache, fever, stiff neck, eye disease, insomnia, ear disease	With needle tip towards orbit of other side 1 to 1.5 cun
Yamen	Between first and second cervical vertebrae, 5 fen above posterior hairline	Deaf-mutism, headache, epilepsy, psychosis	Point towards larynx 1.5 to 2 cun. In pushing needle, soreness, heaviness and distention may be felt. At depth of 2 cun limbs tremble, with shock sensation radiating towards head and neck. Larynx feels heavy. Heavy manipulation may cause dizziness and vomiting.
Zhitong	1.5 cun below yifeng	Toothache	Perpendicularly 0.5 to 1 cun.

Point	Location	Indications	Method
Jiache	At prominence of masseter muscle when tightly clamping teeth together. Finger width above angle of mandible.	Toothache, mandibular arthritis, parotitis, facial paralysis	Perpendicularly 5 *fen* or obliquely to pierce *dicang* point.
Biantao-xian (Dong-feng)	5 *fen* medial to mandibular angle	Tonsillitis, pharyngolaryngitis	Perpendicularly towards tonsil 1 to 1.5 *cun*.
Shang-lian-quan	1 *cun* below mandible	Muteness, profuse salivation, paralysis of hypoglossal nerve	Perpendicularly towards root of tongue 1.5 to 2 *cun*.
Tiantu	At centre of suprasternal fossa	Asthma, coughing, profuse sputum, aphagia	Obliquely at 45 degree angle to sternum for 1 to 1.5 *cun*
Shan-zhong	Between nipples, level with fourth intercostal space.	Asthma, galactozemia, stuffiness, chest pain, intercostal neuralgia	Transversely 0.5 to 1 *cun*
Zhong-wan	4 *cun* above navel, at mid-point of line between navel and xyphoid process	Gastroptosis, epigastric pain, belching, poor appetite	Perpendicularly 1 to 4 *cun*
Tianshu	2 *cun* lateral to navel	Abdominal distention, abdominal pain, vomiting and diarrhoea, constipation, dysentery, ascariasis	Perpendicularly 1 to 2 *cun*
Qihai	1.5 *cun* below navel	Anuria, enuresis, abdominal pain, impotence, menalgia, amenorrhea	Perpendicularly 1.5 to 2 *cun*

Zhixie	2.5 cun below navel	Diarrhoea	Perpendicularly 1.5 to 2 cun
Guanyuan	3 cun below navel	Anuria, enuresis, amenorrhea, menalgia, abdominal pain, enteritis, impotence, prolapse of uterus	Perpendicularly 1.5 to 2 cun
Zhongji	4 cun below navel	Same as above	Perpendicularly 1.5 to 2 cun
Weibao	6 cun lateral to guanyuan point	Prolapse of uterus	Obliquely towards groin 2 to 3 cun
Dazhui	Between spinous processes of seventh cervical and first thoracic vertebra	Acute fever, malaria, bronchitis, hepatitis, epilepsy	Perpendicularly 5 to 8 fen
Dingchuan (Chuanxi)	5 fen lateral to dazhui point	Bronchial asthma, coughing	Obliquely towards vertebral body for 1 cun
Zhiyang	Below seventh thoracic vertebra	Hepatitis, cholecystitis, intercostal neuralgia	Obliquely 5 to 8 fen
Danshu	1.5 cun lateral to and below tenth thoracic vertebra	Acute and chronic hepatitis, cholecystitis	Obliquely downward 0.5 to 1 cun
Mingmen	Just below spinous process of second thoracic vertebra	Lumbago, enuresis, endometritis	Perpendicularly 0.5 to 1 cun
Weishu	1.5 cun lateral to lower margin of twelfth thoracic vertebra	Stomachache, lumbago and backache, insomnia	Perpendicularly 1 to 1.5 cun

Point	Location	Indications	Method
Shenshu	1.5 *cun* lateral to *mingmen* point	Nephritis, lumbago, enuresis, emission, impotence, tinnitus	Perpendicularly 1 to 1.5 *cun*; moxa cylinder or indirect moxibustion
Shiqizhui	Just below fifth lumbar vertebra (inter lumbarsacral joints)	Lumbago, menalgia	Perpendicularly 2 to 2.5 *cun*
Huatojiaji	5 *fen* lateral to vertebrae from first thoracic to first lumbar vertebra	Pain in paraspinal region, intercostal neuralgia, sciatica	Towards vertebral body 1 to 1.5 *cun*
Changqiang	5 *fen* below tip of coccyx	Epilepsy, piles, prolapse of anus, neuralgia of waist	Puncturing 0.5 to 1 *cun*
Huantiao	At lateral third of line connecting coccyx and greater trochanter of thigh bone	Paralysis of lower limb, sciatica, arthritis of hip joint	Deep puncturing towards external genitalia 2 to 3 *cun*
Jianyu	The anterior depression when raising arm	Pain in arm, neck, and back, paralysis	Perpendicularly 1 to 3 *cun*
Sanjiaoji	At centre of deltoid muscle	Pain in shoulder, hemiplegia, shoulder arthritis	Perpendicularly 1 to 2 *cun*
Quchi	At external end of cubital crease when elbow flexed	Antipyresis, decrease in WBC, pain in elbows and arms, toothache, paralysis of upper limbs, lowering blood pressure	Perpendicularly 1 to 3 *cun*
Zhigou	1 *cun* above *waiguan*, 3 *cun* above crease of wrist	Headache, pain in eyes, deafness, pain in elbows and arms, numbness of upper limbs, costal pain, constipation	Perpendicularly 0.5 to 1 *cun* towards *jianshi*

Point	Location	Indications	Method
Waiguan	2 cun above crease of wrist, at lateral end.	Headache, deafness, tinnitus, pain in elbows and arms, numbness of arms	Perpendicularly 0.5 to 1 cun towards opposite neiguan.
Yanglao	On head of ulnar bone where there is a seam when palm turns to face	Pain in elbow or wrist, eye diseases	Perpendicularly 0.3 to 0.5 cun, or towards waiguan for deep puncturing of 0.5 to 1.5 cun
Hegu	At centre of metacarpal bone of index finger	Diseases of head and face, deaf-mutism, pain in arm, numbness of hand, hemiplegia, common cold	Deep puncturing towards houxi point 1 to 3 cun
Zhongzhu	At depression of fourth and fifth metacarpal bones; metacarpal phalangeal joint when forming loose fist	Stagnant pain in shoulder and back, deaf-mutism, aphasia, pain in fourth and fifth fingers	Perpendicularly obliquely upward 1 to 1.5 cun
Shaoze	On ulnar side of little finger, about 1 fen proximal to corner of nail	Shock, neurotic headache, deafness, galactozemia, mastitis	Puncture 1 fen
Bizhong	At centre of two tendons midway on line connecting centre of palmar crease and cubital crease	Paralysis of upper limb	Perpendicularly 1 to 2 cun
Jianshi	1 cun above neiguan	Angina pectoris, palpitation, stomachache, nausea, vomiting, psychosis, malaria.	Perpendicularly 0.8 to 1.2 cun

Luozhen	At point between second and third metacarpal bones, 5 *fen* behind metacarpal-phalangeal joint, back of palm.	Stiffness of neck due to awkward position of neck when sleeping	Perpendicularly 5 *fen*
Neiguan	2 cun above wrist crease, between two tendons	Chest pain, angina pectoris, sore throat, pain in medial side of arm, nausea, vomiting, psychosis	Perpendicularly 0.5 to 1 *cun*
Shenmen	At depression of wrist crease, ulnar side, palmar surface	Neurasthenia, insomnia, hysteria	Perpendicularly 0.3 to 5 *fen*
Yatong	1 *cun* from palm crease between third and fourth metacarpal bones	Toothache	Perpendicularly 5 *fen*
Sifeng	At centre of creases of middle segments of index, middle, ring and little fingers	Dyspepsia in children, emaciation, asthmatic coughing	Puncture 1 *fen* or spot puncture to let out blood with 3-edged needle
Lieque	Above the styloid process of radius, 1.5 *cun* above the transverse crease of wrist	Pain in head and neck, coughing, sore throat, stiff neck, toothache, numbness of upper limb	Pointing tip of needle towards elbow at depth of 0.3 to 0.5 *cun*
Houxi	Clench loose fist; at distal side of crease, small head of fifth metacarpal bone	Pain in extremities, pain at apex of head, lumbago, chest pain, deaf-mutism, psychosis	Perpendicularly 5 *fen* to 1 *cun*

181

Shixuan	At tip of each finger, 2 *fen* from nail	For critical treatment, syncope, heatstroke	Spot puncturing for blood-letting with 3-edged needle.
Yinmen	At centre of *weizhong* and midway in buttock crease	Lumbago, pain in legs, backache, paralysis of lower limbs	Perpendicularly 1 to 3 *cun*
Weizhong	Midpoint of popliteal fossa crease	Backache, lumbago, paralysis of lower limb, erysipelas of leg	Perpendicularly 1 to 3 *cun*
Chengshan	Depression at centre of calf with reverse "V" crease	Spasm of calf, pain of piles, prolapse of anus	Perpendicularly 1 to 3 *cun*
Fengshi	On side of thigh, 7 *cun* above knee, at tip of middle finger when standing erect with arms dropped naturally	Lumbago and pain in leg, paralysis of lower limb	Perpendicularly 1 to 3 *cun*
Xuehai	At point 2 *cun* above lateral margin of patella	Pain in knee, German measles, irregular menses, pain in urethra	Perpendicularly 1 to 2 *cun*
Yanglingquan	At depression anterior and inferior to small head of fibula.	Chest and flank pain, cholecystitis, lumbago, constipation	Slightly obliquely downward 1 to 3 *cun*
Zusanli	3 *cun* below knee, at lateral margin of tibia	Gastrointestinal disease, pain in knee, paralysis of lower limb, goiter, appendicitis	Perpendicularly 1 to 3 *cun*
Dannangxue Lanweixue	1 to 2 *cun* below *yanglingquan*, at tender point	Cholecystitis, chest pain, costal pain, lumbago, pain in legs	Perpendicularly 1 to 3 *cun*

	Location	Indications	Method
yan	Tender point 2 *cun* below *zusanli*	Appendicitis, gastroenteritis, pain in leg	Perpendicularly 1 to 3 *cun*
Xiyan	Depressions at sides of patella bone	Pain in knee joint	Perpendicularly 1 to 3 *cun*
Longzhong	3 *cun* below small head of fibula	Deafness	Perpendicularly 1 to 3 *cun*
Xinfutu	5 *fen* lateral to *futu* point (6 *cun* above external edge of patella)	Exudative arthritis, knee arthralgia	Perpendicularly 1 to 3 *cun*
Dingshang	3 *cun* above knee (3 *cun* above upper edge of patella)	Paralysis of lower limbs, knee arthralgia, muscle pain in lower limbs	Perpendicularly 1 to 2 *cun*
Fenglong	8 *cun* above malleolus, 1.5 *cun* at anterior border of tibia, between tibia and fibula bones	Cough and asthma, profuse sputum, headache, dizziness, pain in lower limbs	Perpendicularly 1 to 3 *cun*
Yinlingquan	At depression of medial malleolus of tibia opposite *yanglingquan*	Anuria, incontinence of urine, urine retention, menalgia, impotence, emission, abdominal pain	Perpendicularly 1 to 3 *cun*; also penetrating to *yanglingquan*
Sanyinjiao	3 *cun* above medial malleolus, at posterior border of tibia	Menalgia, irregular menses, enuresis, emission, abdominal pain, insomnia, urgent micturition, frequent urination, pain in lower limbs	Perpendicularly 1 to 3 *cun* also penetration to *juegu*
Fuliu	2 *cun* above *taixi* point	Profuse sweating, insomnia, edema, sore throat, impotence, enuresis	Perpendicularly 1 to 2 *cun*

Juegu (Xuan-zhong)	3 cun above lateral malleolus	Lumbago, pain in leg, paralysis of lower limbs, pain in shoulder resulting in inability to raise arm.	Perpendicularly 1 to 3 cun; also penetration to sanyinjiao point
Kunlun	Point between heel and lateral malleolus	Lumbago, pain in leg, shoulder pain, stiff neck, pain in ankle joint, hastening of parturition, thyroid disease	Perpendicularly towards medial side for 1 cun, or obliquely penetrating to kunlun point for 1 to 1.5 cun
Taixi	Point between heel and medial malleolus	Insomnia, nephritis, sore throat, impotence, lumbago, backache, pain in ankle, edema enuresis, emission, manalgia	Perpendicularly towards qiuxu for 1 to 3 cun or obliquely 1 to 1.5 cun to kunlun point.
Taichong	1 to 1.5 cun posterior to metatarsal-phalangeal joint, between first and second metatarsal bones	Hypertension, eye diseases, stuffiness, costal pain, dizziness, vertigo, gastrointestinal diseases	Puncture towards ankle for 1 to 1.5 cun
Xingjian	Depression anterior to metatarsal-phalangeal joint, between first and second toes	Hypertension, eye diseases, costal pain, insomnia, hiccup	Puncture towards metatarsal-phalangeal joint to depth of 0.5 to 1 cun
Yong-quan	At depression of sole, between second and third metatarsal bones	For critical use (shock, convulsions, hysteria)	Perpendicularly 0.5 to 1 cun
A'shixue (Tian-ying)	Any point where there is tenderness	Local soreness or numbness	Varies according to condition, commonly 0.5 to 1 cun deep

Cupping Therapy

Cupping is folk therapy widely used in China, first recorded by Ge Hong in his *Prescriptions for Emergency Treatment* in the third century A.D. Burning something in a cup to obtain negative pressure and cupping it onto points of the skin produces vasodilatation and increased volume of blood flow, leading to activation of blood and elimination of stagnation, anti-inflammation and antioncotic action, elimination of wind and dampness. The cups commonly used are made of bamboo, ceramic or glass.

A. Cupping

1. Inner-fire method: With forceps put small ball of cotton soaked in alcohol in cup and let burn for a while. Immediately after removing burning cotton place cup on skin.

2. Light-fire method: Put small ball of cotton in thimble placed on acupoint or place to be cupped. Burn cotton and cover with cup immediately.

3. Drop-fire method: Put piece of burning paper or matchstick into cup. At peak of burning, immediately place cup on skin.

B. Location for cupping (Fig. 271)

Large cups should not be used on chest or abdomen. If chest is injured, the intercostal nerves may be affected, resulting in pain while coughing and difficulty in deep breathing, while injuries caused by such cupping to the thin abdominal wall may suck the intestine with the wall into the cup, resulting in intestinal obstruction or even necrosis.

C. Duration of cupping

A cupping session may last fifteen to twenty mi-

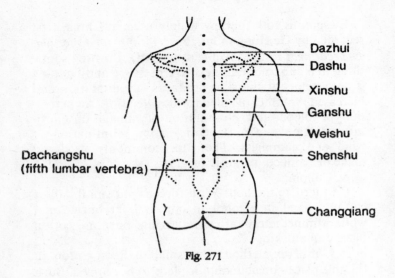

Dazhui

Dashu

Xinshu

Ganshu

Weishu

Shenshu

Dachangshu
(fifth lumbar vertebra)

Changqiang

Fig. 271

nutes, every other day. A course of therapy includes fifteen sessions. To release the cup, gently press skin beside cup to let air into cup, and cup can be removed easily. In case skin is injured, apply local antiseptic.

D. Indications

Angina pectoris (*dazhui, xinshu, ganshu* points), one cup for each point for a total of six cups; hypertension (*dazhui, xinshu, zusanli*); insomnia (put six cups between *dazhui* point and fifth lumbar vertebra one hour before going to bed); acute and chronic bronchitis, acute and chronic pneumonia, whooping cough (*feishu, xinshu, geshu*), six cups in total; headache (*taiyang, dazhui*); malaria (*dazhui*); asthma (*fei-*

shu, xinshu and *geshu*); acute and chronic gastritis, acute and chronic enteritis (*pishu, shenshu, dachangshu*); chronic hepatitis (cupping back in liver region); chronic nephritis, chronic pyelonephritis (in both kidney regions); spasm of diaphragm (*geshu*).

E. Points to remember: Don't use cupping for hemorrhagic disease, edema, emaciation and places where hair is long.

Bloodletting

There are two kinds of bloodletting, venous bloodletting and acupoint bloodletting. The former is commonly used to decrease the total volume of blood so as to lighten the burden on the heart. Moreover, by eliminating stagnant blood, new blood is generated, and as a result, blood stagnation is decreased, viscosity diluted, pressure lowered, and circulation improved. Venous bloodletting also yields diuretic and antitoxic actions. Acupoint bloodletting is commonly used for clearing channels, activating blood and eliminating stasis, as an antipyretic, analgesic and antitoxin, to help regain consciousness, refresh the brain, reduce hotness and swelling and for critical care. Bloodletting often gets results that cannot be obtained through drug therapy.

Venous Bloodletting

A 50 ml sterilized syringe is appropriate. First, draw in 0.5 ml of sterilized sodium citrate as an anticoagulant. Gradually draw 20 to 50 ml blood from the cubital vein. This method is good for critical care of the following diseases.

Hypertensive encephalopathy

Intermittant spasms of the cerebral vessels are a result of hypertension. Manifestations are headache, dizziness, vertigo, numbness of the extremities or even temporary paralysis, aphasia and blindness, which may last for several minutes or even several days. Severe and persistent cerebral vascular spasm may cause sudden and severe rise of blood pressure, accompanied by severe headache, vomiting, convulsions and coma, leading to acute circulatory disturbance, cerebral edema and increase of cranial pressure.

By venous bloodletting of 20 to 50 ml of blood, most of the above symptoms may disappear. Depressors or drugs for activating blood and eliminating stasis administered following the bloodletting will yield quite satisfactory results. However, it is advisable not to lower the blood pressure too much in a patient suffering a long hypertension, since the patient will not be able to adapt and may run the risk of cerebral thrombosis or coronary thrombosis.

Hypertension crisis

This disorder refers to a sudden severe rise of blood pressure with symptoms of headache, nausea, vomiting, blurring of vision, or even coma, convulsions, dyspnea, palpitation or pulmonary edema in severe cases. All the manifestations are quite similar to those for hypertensive encephalopathy except there is no paralysis.

For emergency treatment, 20 to 50 ml of blood are let, followed by a depressor such as a depressor tablet of chrysanthemum, vasodepressor compound tablet, hydralazine.

Points to remember: same as above.

Uremia due to acute nephritis and toxemia during pregnancy.

These are common severe disorders, and their treatment is, of course, of great importance. Main symptoms are intractable headache, increase of blood pressure, nausea, vomiting, palpitation, edema, dizziness, etc.

A bloodletting of 30 to 50 ml will relieve nausea, vomiting, headache and dizziness and lower blood pressure.

Local edema

Also known as angio neurotic edema. Edema of the larynx may result in fatal asphyxiation.

For critical care, 10 to 20 ml of bloodletting will relieve laryngeal edema.

Pulmonary edema

This is the result of pulmonary blood stagnation, manifested by extreme difficulty in breathing, orthopnea, hemoptysis with foamy and serious sputum. It is fatal if no emergency care is given.

For emergency treatment, 20 to 30 ml of blood should be let; dyspnea will be decreased greatly. Cupping of the *feishu*, *xinshu* and *geshu* points with large cups for fifteen minutes will give even more satisfactory results.

Cardiac asthma

Often seen in a rheumatic heart disease or hypertensive heart disease. The disease often manifests a sudden onset of stuffiness, dyspnea, palpitation and wheezing. It is fatal if no emergency care is given.

For critical care, 20 to 50 ml of blood are let, together with injection of 0.25 gm of aminophylline. Asthma can be relieved immediately and edema lessened, thus relieving the cardiac burden. The treatment also yields diuretic and antitoxic effects.

Cardiac type of beriberi

This is the result of a severe deficiency of vitamin B1. It often has a sudden onset, with marked palpitation, dyspnea, stuffiness, vomiting, thirst, anuria, and cyanosis of nails, lips and face. The patient is in an extremely critical condition.

For emergency treatment, 20 to 30 ml of blood are let to promptly alleviate the symptoms. Intramuscular injection of vitamin B1 yields remarkable effects. It should be emphasized that there are two kinds of vitamin B1 injections; one can be injected intravenously, the other cannot. Application of the wrong type would prove fatal to the patient.

Remarks: For anaemia and heart failure bloodletting is prohibited. It is also inadvisable for uraemia due to severe dehydration, hemorrhage, shock in peripheral and tuberculosis of kidneys.

Acupoint Bloodletting

Useful for the following disorders:

Acute tonsillitis

The tonsils redden and swell when inflamed producing sore throat, difficulty in deglutition and profuse saliva secretion.

For treatment, palpate the inflamed tonsil with clean right middle finger to determine whether there is undulation. An incision for discharging pus is necessary in case of undulation. If the tonsil feels hard without undulation, acupuncture of the internal and external *shuliao* point is indicated (in the middle of nasal septum). Seven to eight drops of blood are let. The swollen tonsil will shrink within ten minutes, and deglutition will no longer be difficult. The effect is wonderful. After that, "paste for nourishing vital essence and clearing the lungs" is administered.

Acute gastroenteritis

The onset is sudden, beginning with nausea and vomiting, followed by abdominal ache and diarrhoea with watery and stinking stool several times or some ten times a day. The stool may be mixed with mucus and blood. Vomiting may also appear several or a dozen times a day. At first, food residue is vomited, followed by bile. No fever can be detected in mild cases. However, dehydration, acidosis or even shock may be observed in severe cases.

For treatment, puncture the *quze* point with a sterilized three-edged needle and let one or two drops of blood. Vomiting may be cured. Needling of the *weizhong* point to bleed has an antidiarrhoea effect, while bleeding the *shuliao* point is effective for stopping vomiting and restlessness.

Malaria

This is an infectious disease caused by plasmodium protozoa with manifestations of periodic cold tremors followed by a high fever of 40 degrees centigrade, restlessness, thirst, profuse perspiration, etc.

For critical treatment, cupping and acupuncture two hours before the onset of symptoms should be administered. Bloodletting of the *dazhui* point with a sterilized three-edged needle for one or two drops of blood is followed by fifteen minutes of cupping with a middle-size cup. Then oral administration of *Fructus Bruceae*, ten to fifteen capsules three times daily after meals. After the illness is under control, the drug should be continued for two days at half the previous dosage for consolidation of efficacy.

Heat stroke

Mild cases manifest headache, dizziness, stuffiness, nausea, fever, thirst and weakness, while severe cases manifest headache, nausea, vomiting, profuse sweating, restlessness, sudden coma, convulsions and unconsciousness.

For emergency treatment of comatous cases, puncture the *renzhong, hegu* and *shixuan* points with three-edged needles for spot bleeding. Administer orally twenty "pills of infinity" (*wuji* pills) (lesser for children). Take cold drinks to achieve quick results.

About the Author

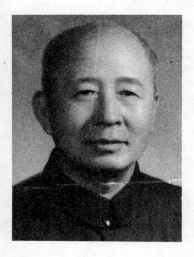

Born in 1910, Professor Hu Bin, head physician of the Department of Breathing Exercises, Academy of Traditional Chinese Medicine, graduated from Xinjing Medical University (now Jilin Medical University) in 1938. He has been director of Fuyu County Hospital, Jilin Province; head of the Internal Medicine Department of Red Cross Hospital, Changchun City, Jilin Province; director of the Department of Internal Medicine, Provincial Hospital of Zhangjiakou City, Qahar Province (now Hebei Province); member of the Academic Committee, Academy of Traditional Chinese Medicine, and head of the Department of Internal Medicine, Beijing Traditional Chinese Medicine Hospital.

In his forties, Professor Hu suffered from neurasthenia, high blood pressure and coronary heart disease. He was also suffering from hepatitis, arteriosclerosis and functional disturbances of the sympathetic nervous system. Adept in pathology, Professor Hu studied the traditional rehabilitation medicine of ancient China. By applying comprehensive therapy, including breathing exercises, shadow boxing and slapping exercises, assisted by drug remedies, he successfully and effectively conquered all these chronic ailments. Now he is in his seventh decade, full of energy, with a high complexion and facile imagination.

In 1964 the task of conquering high blood pressure and coronary heart disease was given to the traditional Chinese medicine (TCM) workers by the Ministry of Public Health, and the academy where Dr. Hu worked was appointed for its accomplishment. Through practice on 115 cases of high blood pressure and 65 cases of coronary heart disease Dr. Hu was able to cure the ailments by comprehensive therapy in 90 percent of the cases, to relieve symptoms and to consolidate the treatment efficacy.

Combining traditional Chinese and Western medicine, Dr. Hu has engaged in the clinical study of cardiovascular diseases over a period of some fifty years. He has conscientiously studied a large quantity of ancient medical literature as well as widespread folk medicine. Thus he has accumulated rich practical experience in both traditional Chinese and Western medicine and is expert in the following: treatment of coronary heart disease, cerebral arteriosclerosis and cerebral thrombosis by activating blood circulation and eliminating stagnation; treatment of sphenoid hyperplasia and hemiplegia by activating blood circulation, eliminating stagnation, softening hard lumps, and dredging the channels and collaterals; treatment of chronic hepatitis, chronic nephritis and chronic gastritis by activating blood circulation, eliminating stagnation, clearing heat, subsiding inflammation and detoxifying; the influence of deficiency of the kidney on body health and its convalescent measures as well as every field of traditional Chinese methods of rehabilitation medicine, such as breathing exercises.

Dr. Hu has already published some fifty academic as well as popular articles on health care and internal medicine. His monographs include "An Introduction to the Science of Breathing Exercises," "Clinical Treatment of Internal Diseases in Traditional Chinese Medicine," "Prevention and Treatment of High Blood Pressure and Coronary Heart Disease," "Selected Collections of Treating Malignant Tumours with Chinese Herbs" and "Clinical Experience of Integrating Traditional Chinese and Western Medicine."

Traditional Chinese Therapeutic Exercises and Techniques

Atlas of Therapeutic Motion for Treatment and Health
—A Guide to Traditional Chinese Massage and Exercise Therapy

Traditional Chinese Therapeutic Exercises
Standing Pole

Chinese Single Broadsword
A Primer of Basic Skills and Performance Routines for Practitioners

14-Series Sinew-Transforming Exercises

Infantile *Tuina* Therapy

Eating Your Way to Health
Dietotherapy in Traditional Chinese Medicine

Keep Fit the Chinese Way

Meridian Qigong

Taiji Qigong
Twenty-eight Steps

The Mystery of Longevity

图书在版编目(CIP)数据

中国传统的康复医学:英文/胡斌著.—北京:
外文出版社,1991(1995年重印)
ISBN 7－119－00908－7

Ⅰ.中… Ⅱ.胡… Ⅲ.康复医学—中国—英文 Ⅳ.R49

中国版本图书馆 CIP 数据核字 (95) 第 13843 号

中国传统的康复医学

胡 斌 著

*

© 外文出版社

外文出版社出版
(中国北京百万庄路 24 号)
邮政编码 100037
北京外文印刷厂印刷
中国国际图书贸易总公司发行
(中国北京车公庄西路 35 号)
北京邮政信箱第 399 号　邮政编码 100044
1991 年(34 开)第一版
1995 年第二次印刷
(英)
ISBN 7－119－00908－7 /R·21(外)
01180
14－E－2238P